TREATING CHILDHOOD AND ADOLESCENT ANXIETY

A GUIDE FOR CAREGIVERS

ELI R. LEBOWITZ · HAIM OMER

WILEY

Library of Congress Cataloging-in-Publication Data:

Lebowitz, Eli R.
    Treating childhood and adolescent anxiety : a guide for caregivers / Eli R. Lebowitz
and Haim Omer.
       pages   cm
    Includes bibliographical references and index.
    ISBN 978-1-118-12101-6 (hbk. : alk. paper); ISBN 978-1-118-26275-7 (ebk);
    ISBN 978-1-118-23802-8 (ebk); ISBN 978-1-118-22469-4 (ebk)
    1. Anxiety in children.   2. Anxiety in adolescence.   3. Anxiety–Treatment.
I. Omer, Haim.   II. Title.
    BF723.A5L393 2013
    618.92'852206—dc23
                                                                    2012048965

I dedicate this book to Sergeant Zeev Buzaglo, a fearless young man whose smile could make anyone brave.

—ERL

I dedicate this book to all the people who helped me live better with my own fears.

—HO

I fear not might
Nor weather's blight
But the daily death of night

Not confrontation
Condemnation
But your salty accusation

I fear not arrow, sword or spear
But you do. Making distant near
And all I truly fear, is fear

Contents

PART THREE: WORKING WITH PARENTS

PART FOUR: ANCILLARY ISSUES

Preface

WHY ANOTHER BOOK ON ANXIETY?

There are quite a few good books about children's anxiety. There are also excellent manuals for the treatment of anxious children, which do a great job of presenting what have become accepted standards of treatment in the field of pediatric anxiety. So, one question in setting out to write a guide for caregivers working with fearful children and their parents is: What for? Why go to the effort of creating one more book? And, no less compellingly, why would anyone buy this book rather than the others that have come before?

In the end, the answer to this question has been the same one that guides much of the work that we and our colleagues do in the search for ways to help the families of children suffering from anxiety. It comes down to the troubling fact that although the treatments that are available today are helpful for many, perhaps even a majority, of these children — many are still left unaided. As psychologists, psychiatrists, and caregivers in the field of childhood anxiety disorders, we pride ourselves on the ability to effectively help many. But a substantial minority, probably around a third, is still crying out for us to try harder. And when we're talking about anxiety in children, one third is a great many kids.

So although one important part of this book covers territory that has become familiar to at least some of the professionals, and even many of the parents who through circumstances have become lay experts in the field of anxiety, other parts chart newer and more exciting waters.

Rather than being satisfied with presenting the state of the art, we are trying to show the state of some of tomorrow's art.

INTEGRATING THE INDIVIDUAL AND THE FAMILY

An unfortunate accident of history is the divide that has traditionally existed between family-oriented therapists and theoreticians, who view a child's disorder as the manifestation of a systemic family problem, and most others in the field of child mental health. The paradigm that has dominated psychiatry and clinical psychology for much of its history has been more individually focused—treating the child with only little attention paid to familial factors. This is unfortunate because the absence of cross-fertilization of ideas and skills has hampered the development of treatment models that straddle the gulf, benefiting from and adding to the knowledge of each.

This kind of integration could be helpful in most disorders of childhood, but nowhere is it more needed, or its absence more glaring, than in the context of anxiety disorders. At their very heart anxiety disorders are interpersonal and systemic in nature. Yet a child's disorder is also an individual feature of that child. Some problems exist encapsulated within the individual suffering from them. If a child has a dental cavity, for example, that problem exists in his mouth. If a child has flat feet the problem lives in her shoes. However, when a child suffers from anxiety the problem exists both within the child and in the interpersonal space of the relationship between parent and child. As we discuss in depth in the second half of this book, parents, to whom children look for protection when they feel threatened, are intricately caught up in the disorder of a child who experiences chronic threat.

Throughout this book we attempt to integrate the individual and family perspectives, learning from both and offering strategies that stem from this assimilation. This is particularly true of the *SPACE Program* manual presented in the third part of this book. The SPACE Program, or Supportive Parenting for Anxious Childhood Emotions, is a treatment protocol for childhood anxiety and obsessive compulsive disorder. However, it is a completely parent-based intervention. The integration of a family perspective with the knowledge and experience that have been gained in the past decades in the treatment of anxiety is what make this treatment possible. One of the most exciting features of this kind of novel intervention is in allowing us to treat children who may be unresponsive or resistant to individual child-based cognitive behavioral therapy.

Another benefit of an approach informed by both individual and family perspectives is the ability to cast fathers and mothers of anxious children in a much more active role in aiding their own children. Seeing your children suffering is terribly hard, and so is seeing their function and development impaired by emotional challenges. But the feelings of helplessness caused by watching the struggles without having a role in helping to overcome those difficulties can make the experience much worse. When we are able to guide parents toward more active roles and empower them with the feeling of being part of the solution to their child's distress, we are actually already making things better—even before symptoms ever improve. Helplessness leads to despair and frustration, where a sense of purpose can lend hope and self-efficacy.

Another example of the integration of family and individual perspectives is the chapter on *adult entitled dependence*. Grown children who, for a variety of reasons, have not successfully separated from home and parents and continue to rely on them to a high degree are a growing problem around the world. Despite this there is a dearth of treatment strategies for addressing these intractable situations. Adopting an integrated approach opens up novel strategies for helping families to create change and momentum in otherwise stagnant situations. Yet another example on which we bring the integration to bear is that of *school refusal*, a common problem that inherently involves both child and parents and often appears mired in conflict and insusceptible to traditional approaches.

Lest anyone mistake our integration of familial and parental factors into the conceptualization and treatment of childhood anxiety for a return to the unmissed days of 'parent blaming,' let us be clear. We do not believe that parents are to blame for their children's disorders. The notion of blaming parents for their children's anxiety is as alien to us as the idea of them being irrelevant is foreign. We do not hold parents responsible for a child's anxiety but we believe most parents are affected by their children's disorder and that most parents long to be able to help their child to overcome adversity. By recognizing the systemic nature of pediatric anxiety, we are moving away from a choice between parents as irrelevant bystanders or parents as flawed and at fault. Rather we cast parents in the role of supporters and leaders and provide therapists with the tools to guide parents in helping their children to overcome anxiety and lead happier, healthier lives.

In short, it is our hope that this book informs both caregivers and caretakers, offering practical, evidence-based, and theory-driven strategies for helping children to overcome anxiety in its many forms.

—Eli Lebowitz

Introduction

CHAPTER ONE

Anxiety Disorders of Children and Adolescents

Anxiety disorders are common in children and adolescents and can impact many aspects of healthy functioning and development. Anxiety disorders in children also impact parents and family.

Key points in this chapter:

- The prevalence and course of anxiety disorders.
- The different anxiety disorders and the criteria for their diagnosis.
- The impact these disorders can have on the child and the family.
- The role of primary care providers.

COMMON ANXIETY DISORDERS OF CHILDHOOD AND ADOLESCENCE

Anxiety disorders are the most frequent disorders of childhood, and likely of adulthood as well (Kessler, Chiu, Demler, & Walters, 2005). Lifetime and point prevalence estimates of their occurrence range quite widely, with the lowest estimates indicating a rate of around 3% for at least one anxiety disorder at any given time and the highest estimates indicating that upward of 30% (Costello, Egger, & Angold; Merikangas et al., 2010) of people will suffer from an anxiety disorder at some point in their lives. The differences in estimates reported likely stem from the different populations studied, the different tools used for screening and assessment, the variability in criteria and procedures for establishing diagnoses (for instance, *child only* versus *child or parent* report), the quality of sampling in different studies, and other methodological variables. In any event, there can be little doubt that anxiety disorders are common among children.

Suffering from anxiety can have a devastating and widespread impact on a child and on the family. Anxiety disorders tend to be chronic (Keller et al., 1992), rarely "just going away" on their own with spontaneous remission in only a minority of cases. But the impact of the anxiety extends beyond the specific criteria used for establishing a diagnosis (Angold et al., 1998). Physical and mental health, social functioning, academic achievement, family relationships, and overall quality of life can all be negatively affected by anxiety (Woodward & Fergusson, 2001).

The current version of the *Diagnostic and Statistical Manual of the American Psychiatric Association* (*DSM-IV-TR*) (American Psychiatric Association, 2000) recognizes the existence of a number of discrete patterns of anxiety-related symptoms and this is to be the case in the upcoming *DSM-V* as well, despite some changes (e.g., excluding obsessive-compulsive disorder from the anxiety disorders group). In this book, however, we have chosen to discuss the anxiety disorders as a group, including OCD, for a number of reasons.

First, the categorization of anxiety disorders into separate entities relies primarily on identifying different stimuli or situations that provoke the anxiety and classifying the disorder accordingly. For example, those who respond with anxiety to social situations are likely to meet criteria for social phobia whereas children who have a fear of separation from their parents would better be described as having separation anxiety disorder. Although such a classification serves a number of important purposes, such as comparing the prevalence or treatment responsiveness of particular patterns of fear, it also creates a certain illusion—the idea that the problem is actually closely tied to the particular stimulus the individual fears. In this book we take the approach that anxiety disorders are more closely connected to how a child manages fear and the experience of anxiety than it is to the specific things that trigger the anxiety.

Additionally, the high rates of comorbidity between anxiety disorders support the idea that an underlying difficulty in regulating anxiety is a helpful way of conceptualizing the problem. Clinical experience, epidemiological studies, and the multitude of clinical samples reported on in papers about anxiety point to the conclusion that having one anxiety disorder is a powerful predictor of actually meeting criteria for at least one more (Rapee, Schniering, & Hudson, 2009). Both longitudinal and retrospective studies show that although anxiety tends to be chronic within disorders, having one anxiety disorder today also predicts having another different one in the future (Bittner, 2007). Although the theoretical implications of the high rates of comorbidity are equivocal (see Curry, March, & Hervey, 2004), they support considering all the subcategories of anxiety as a group.

Another reason for treating anxiety disorders as a group rather than as separate entities is the similarity in proven effective treatments. Using the statistical methodology of analysis of variance as a metaphor, one might say that the within group differences in treating anxiety are rather more pronounced than between group differences. In other words, treating a child or adolescent with anxiety is similar across disorders, although it may vary significantly between specific children. Two children suffering from social phobia might be no more similar in the course of therapy than a child with social phobia and one with a specific phobia, although some details of the treatment will naturally vary.

Finally, much of the work with anxious children requires addressing the whole family's needs and roles. Parents of anxious children are faced with similar dilemmas, challenges, and questions although their children may experience the fear in different situations (Lebowitz, Woolston, et al., 2012). The questions that are raised by parents, such as "Should I give in or demand that he does it?"; "When is accommodation a good thing and when is it a problem?"; or "Is this a serious problem or simply attention-seeking behavior?" cut across the spectrum of anxiety disorders, ignoring nosological categories.

The following section describes the different anxiety disorders diagnosable under *DSM-IV-TR* and the way they affect the child and family. Later chapters focus on individual and family models and treatment strategies that can be applied across the range of disorders. Though there are many specific manuals for various disorders, and new ones are likely to appear, here we draw from the best-known techniques to date to help clinicians, parents, and children facing any of these disorders.

Separation Anxiety Disorder

This is the only anxiety disorder still classified in *DSM-IV* as a disorder of childhood, indicating the acknowledgment that anxiety is generally quite similar in its manifestations at different ages, although specific criteria can vary for diagnosing children in other disorders as well. Indeed, in the upcoming *DSM-V*, separation anxiety disorder is to be moved from the section on disorders of childhood and placed with all other anxiety disorders.

Separation anxiety is characterized by a child's fear of separation from the home or caretakers. Children with separation anxiety usually worry about bad things that could happen to them or to their parents during times of separation. For example, children might fear being kidnapped or getting hurt when a parent is not there to help them. Children who worry about things that could happen to their parents might imagine them getting into a car accident or some such disaster. For some children the fear will be that the parents might simply disappear and never return, and they might spend time fantasizing about being reunited with their parents, even during minor separations.

Children with separation anxiety will often object to or try to avoid even small periods of separation, and some might strive to maintain direct contact with parents whenever possible. Many children with separation anxiety will even follow their parents from room to room around the house. A special focus for many children with separation anxiety is bedtime, when they may feel afraid of being left alone in their room and prefer to sleep next to a parent, either in their own bed or in the parents'. Some children will report having nightmares in which they are separated from their parents. Another night-related separation fear is that of being awake after parents are asleep. Many children try to avoid this either by going to bed first or by demanding that their parents stay up until they are asleep.

Many children will exhibit manifest anxiety by begging not to be left alone, clinging to a parent's legs or even trying to block the door of the house when parents want to leave. Some might repeatedly try to make contact with the parents during times of separation, for example, by phoning them endlessly through the day. A major concern for some children with separation anxiety is the separation caused by the need to go to school and school avoidance is a common outcome of the fear. Others may go to school but find it hard to focus on classwork because of their persistent worrying.

Not surprisingly, separation anxiety is most common in younger children and tends to decrease in prevalence as children enter and pass through adolescence, although separation anxiety in young adults is also encountered. When a child with separation anxiety is absent from school for extended periods of time, the likelihood that they will continue to suffer from the disorder in adulthood increases. Early onset is specified in the diagnosis if the disorder appears before age 6, but the natural tendency of young children to proximity with their parents must be taken into account.

Separation anxiety has the clear potential to disrupt both the child's individual functioning; for example, by limiting school attendance and performance or by curtailing social activities (e.g., avoiding sleepovers or visits to peers), as well as family functioning. Siblings may find themselves accommodating the child's anxiety; for example, by spending less time with parents because of their need to be with the anxious child. Parents often adapt to the child's anxiety by limiting their own departures from the home, returning earlier than they otherwise would from work, or sleeping alongside the child.

Panic Disorder and Agoraphobia

Panic attacks are brief periods of time during which a child, despite the absence of immediate danger, experiences intense anxious arousal. The panic attack can be primarily physiological in nature, including symptoms such as sweating, racing heart, shortness of breath, trembling, chest pain, or feelings of choking. In other cases the panic attacks have a more cognitive focus, including terrifying thoughts about losing control or going crazy, fear of dying, or feeling like reality has "shifted" (derealization), or that they have become detached from themselves (depersonalization). For many children the attack includes both cognitive and physiological symptoms.

Panic disorder is characterized by the presence of repeated panic attacks and a persistent worry about the possibility of having more such attacks in the future. Although the attacks themselves are brief, typically peaking within 10 or 15 minutes and even though some children experience only few actual attacks, they can be severely impaired by the fear of the experience being repeated. In addition, many children suffering from panic disorder report having frequent physical signs of anxiety that do not reach the level of a panic attack but cause discomfort or make them worry that an attack is imminent. This may be due to a tendency to constantly monitor their own inner physiological state (Schmidt, Lerew, & Trakowski, 1997), leading them to focus on transient normal changes that would otherwise not receive any attention.

Another theory proposes that the symptoms of panic are caused by an unnecessary triggering of the body system usually active during potential suffocation, as happens during overexposure to carbon dioxide (Klein, 1993). Children who have panic disorder may also interpret normal physical discomfort such as a headache or stomachache as the sign of something catastrophic, such as a life-threatening illness. This kind of monitoring and misinterpretation can lead to a vicious cycle in which focusing on their body causes them to recognize any changes, which in turn heightens anxiety. This can lead to a panic attack and causes even more inner focus and monitoring. Children may ask their parents to check their pulse, listen to their hearts, or provide reassurance that they are well. A related fear in children exists when a child is very afraid of vomiting and begins to focus on internal gastrointestinal signs, searching for clues of impending need to vomit (although this would be diagnosed as a specific phobia rather than panic disorder).

In many cases panic disorder will be associated with *agoraphobia*, which describes the fear or avoidance of situations in which they think they may experience symptoms of panic. A child who has had a panic attack in school, for example, may be afraid to go to school because of a fear of having another panic attack while there. In severe cases the avoidance will be generalized to any place outside of the home and the child may refuse to go out at all or need to be accompanied by a parent who can "rescue" them should an attack begin. This pattern increases the potential of even few and brief panic attacks to severely impair a child's well-being and development for lengthy periods of time.

Panic disorder and agoraphobia are more common in adolescents than in children and only a relatively small number of cases are reported in younger children. The diagnosis, however, relies on the existence of at least two episodes that meet criteria for a full-blown panic attack, including at least 4 of the 13 possible symptoms listed by the *DSM-IV-TR*. Episodes including less than four such symptoms (dubbed *limited-symptom attacks*) may be significantly more common in the younger population.

The effect of panic disorder and agoraphobia on the family's and parents' functioning is caused by the need to provide reassurance to a child or even to arrange for repeated medical examinations. These may serve to alleviate parental worry about the child's health but can also be triggered by the child's need of professional medical confirmation that he or she is not at risk. The dramatic manifestation of anxiety, accompanied by terrible thoughts and extreme physical agitation, can cause parents to panic and be overwhelmed by their own fear for the child's health. Parents are often much at a loss regarding how to respond to a child during an attack. The child, seeing how upset and worried the parents are, may take this as confirmation that something is indeed terribly wrong. Agoraphobia can impact the family by limiting the child's ability to function independently, requiring parental accompaniment to locations and activities that would otherwise be done without them.

Specific Phobia

Specific phobias are fears of particular things or situations that cause a child to avoid contact with the feared stimulus or to be distressed when contact must be endured. There is no real limit on the objects that can become the focus of a child's phobia but some common groups of phobias include fear of animals such as snakes, bugs, dogs, or bats; fear of natural phenomena including heights, darkness, storms, and water; fear of blood, injections, and medical procedures; and fears relating to particular situations such as riding in a car, plane, or elevator or of being in closed places. Other common fears in childhood include the fears of clowns, loud noises, or the things that make them such as balloons and the fear of throwing up. Some children will explain their fear as relating to a thought of harm that might come to them through exposure to the phobic object. For example, children might think they would be bitten if they were to approach a dog. Other children will have a fear of their own reaction to the stimulus. For example, the level of horror and revulsion that many children experience when confronted by a spider can be enough to cause the phobia even if they do not believe the spider is dangerous.

Although adults must recognize that their fear is irrational and extreme in order for the diagnosis to be conferred, this requirement does not exist for children. Many children, however, do display this kind of insight and acknowledge that the degree of fear or avoidance is not warranted by the realistic risk. Having insight can facilitate treatment of the phobia as children are more likely to engage in a process meant to reduce the fear if they realize it is not actually protecting them from harm.

Children with phobias will try to avoid any exposure to the feared stimulus. Often they will generalize the fear and avoidance to a wide array of situations, beyond direct contact with the object of their fear. For example, a child with a fear of dogs may be afraid to walk down entire streets because of a fear of seeing a dog or hearing one bark. Or the child might attempt to avoid any contact with pictures, toys, or stories that involve dogs. This pattern of generalization can cause the phobia to have a much wider impact on a child's functioning than might otherwise have been expected. A child with a phobia of sharks might never encounter a shark but be terrified at any contact with water, even in the shower.

Phobias are common across all ages and tend to appear relatively early in childhood (Kessler, Berglund, et al., 2005). However, often the phobias are diagnosed as a comorbid condition while another anxiety disorder was the actual trigger for treatment. This is likely because, unless the phobia is having a particularly detrimental effect on a child's life, many parents assume that phobias are normal and do not require treatment. However, treating a phobia relatively early on can serve both to minimize its impact and the opportunities for greater generalization of avoidance and to provide the child with a model of overcoming fear — replacing coping strategies for avoidance as the response to anxiety.

A child's phobia can impact the family in various ways, including by creating avoidance that the entire family adheres to. For example, one child who had a fear of dogs insisted that the family not rent any movie that featured dogs and would vet (excuse the pun) any selection before allowing it to be rented from a video library. A child with a fear of driving or of traveling over bridges might curtail family activities, or one with a fear of loud noises may be unable to tolerate parties being held at home, even for siblings. Some children become so afraid of insects that they object to any windows being opened in the home, creating a potentially stifling environment.

Social Phobia

Social phobia, also known as *social anxiety disorder*, is characterized by marked and persistent fear of social situations in which the child will be subject to potential scrutiny by others. Children may fear acting in an embarrassing or humiliating way or showing overt symptoms of anxiety such as stammering, blushing, or trembling. The thoughts that are triggered by social situations may include the idea of being perceived as anxious, weak, stupid, or "crazy." Physical symptoms are almost always associated with the anxiety-provoking situations and can include racing heart, tremors, sweating, blushing, gastrointestinal discomfort, and muscle tension. As a consequence, the child may avoid social situations like eating or speaking in public. When children must confront these situations, they usually do so with considerable distress. The avoidance of such situations or the distress they cause can interfere significantly with the normal routine of the individual, their occupational or academic functioning, or their social activities and relationships. Because transient periods of shyness or social awkwardness are normal, particularly in adolescence, children are only diagnosed with social phobia if their symptoms have persisted for at least 6 months.

In some cases the social phobia will be limited to particular situations such as attending parties, speaking in class, or talking to girls. In other cases, however, almost any social interaction can be the trigger for intense fear and the avoidance is very broad. In these cases, termed *generalized social phobia*, the disorder has tremendous potential to disrupt normal development. Some children retreat into almost complete self-isolation, making every effort to avoid all contact with others. This can lead to school avoidance as well as to negative impact on the child's mood and self-esteem. Social phobia, however, does not necessarily indicate a lack of social awareness or of social interest (Brown, Silvia, Myin-Germeys, & Kwapil, 2007; Coplan, Prakash, O'Neil, & Armer, 2004). Many children with even severe social phobia long for friendship or for the ability to interact more confidently with others, even while they may make every effort to avoid doing so.

Social phobia is commonly diagnosed in mid- to late adolescence but often had its onset in much earlier childhood. Younger children who are described as shy or behaviorally inhibited may be later diagnosed with social phobia. In other cases particular incidents or situations might precipitate the onset of social phobia in a person without a pronounced history of shyness. For example, a teenager who is teased because of acne might develop social phobia and be embarrassed to be seen by others. In some children social anxiety might cause them to be ashamed of the need for glasses or braces, leading them to either avoid being seen or to refuse to wear the corrective apparatus.

A rarer but related disorder most commonly diagnosed in young children is *selective mutism*, which is characterized by the failure to speak in some social situations despite speaking in other ones. Children with selective mutism might speak normally at home but refuse to speak outside of the house, or they might speak with family and other children but not with adults. Although not formally part of the diagnosis, selective mutism is commonly associated with shyness and also accompanied by other manifestations of childish anxiety such as clinging to parents in social situations.

Children with social phobia or selective mutism often make use of parents or siblings as mediators and go-betweens for interacting with the social world. Socially shy children might refuse to talk on the telephone and demand that someone else at home speak for them, or they may be too embarrassed to speak with a stranger and have someone else function as their representative. In older children and adolescents particularly, this pattern can cause them to appear more impaired and can limit many age-appropriate functions. In some cases a child with social anxiety will also attempt to limit the entrance of guests or strangers into the home, imposing limitations on parents and siblings.

Obsessive-Compulsive Disorder

Obsessive-compulsive disorder (OCD) is characterized by recurring thoughts, images, or impulses that are intrusive and distressing (obsessions) or by the need to perform repetitive behaviors or adhere to strict behavioral rules (compulsions). Most children with OCD report having both obsessions and compulsions but some will not be able to identify specific thoughts or behaviors. The variety of potential obsessional content or compulsive behaviors is unlimited, but some common obsessions include thoughts about contamination, doubts over whether actions were performed, thoughts relating to distressing aggressive or sexual content, and thoughts about negative things that could happen to the self or to loved ones. Worry about parents dying is a common obsession in children. A particular kind of contamination obsession sometimes seen in children is the fear of being contaminated by another person's personality or by specific traits associated with that person and perceived as undesirable.

Typical compulsions include the need to repeatedly wash hands, the need to perform actions a set number of times, behaviors aimed at producing order or symmetry (in actual objects such as by lining things up on a shelf or in the inner experience such as by touching with the left hand something that was touched with the right hand), and repeatedly checking things (e.g., checking that the water was turned off). The compulsions are usually performed to alleviate distress caused by the obsessions. Although adults must have recognized at some point that the obsessions or compulsions are not reasonable, this kind of insight is not a requirement in children. Insight is associated with age so that younger children often do not display insight whereas adolescents generally do.

Although in many cases the compulsion logically or directly relates to the content of an obsession, for example, when children wash their hands because of an obsession about dirt or germs, this is not always the case. Other children might engage in the same hand-washing behavior because of the thought that if they did not, their parents would suffer a car accident. In many cases the child will attempt to avoid situations that are likely to trigger obsessions or the need to perform compulsions. For example, children with a recurring image of cutting themselves might try to avoid any contact with knives or sharp objects, and others with a fear of contamination might go to great lengths to avoid contact with potential contaminators. In other cases the child will avoid starting a behavior that is likely to become prolonged because of ritualization, for instance, avoiding showering because it is hard to get out of the shower, or avoiding reading because of the need to repeatedly read the same sentence again and again. This avoidant tendency can greatly exacerbate the negative impact of the disorder on daily life.

The onset of the disorder can occur early in childhood, although a later onset is more common. Symptoms usually appear gradually and gain in severity and frequency over time but sometimes severe symptoms can appear suddenly. This may be triggered by particularly anxiety-provoking incidents, such as exposure to distressing content that the child remains mentally focused on. One possible cause of the sudden appearance of OCD symptoms is the syndrome known as PANS (previously PANDAS; (Swedo et al., 1998)) or Pediatric Acute-onset Neuropsychiatric Syndrome (Swedo, Leckman, & Rose, 2012). This is the sudden appearance of obsessive-compulsive symptoms triggered by antibodies produced in response to infections with Group A beta-hemolytic streptococci. However, the sudden appearance of OCD symptoms, even when preceded by strep infection, are not sufficient to establish a diagnosis of PANS, and ancillary symptoms such as changes in motor functioning, mood, and personality or the appearance of separation anxiety and enuresis need to be considered.

OCD has the potential to greatly disrupt the life and development of both the child and the family. The avoidance of potential triggers described earlier, the amounts of time spent on compulsions, the cognitive resources usurped by the disorder, and the distress of feeling out of control with regard to one's own mind can wreak havoc on a child's life, affecting school performance, academic achievement, mood, and general well-being. Many children fear that they are crazy or are deeply ashamed or guilt-ridden because of the content of their intrusive thoughts. Although the disorder is not uncommon, the seeming strangeness of thinking unwanted thoughts or behaving in irrational ways leads most children to be reluctant to discuss the problem with others, sometimes including parents. This can serve to delay the time to treatment as well as to increase a child's loneliness or discouragement.

Parents of children with OCD almost invariably report engaging in accommodating behaviors (see more detail on this in Chapter 3 on family accommodation). Accommodation can include providing reassurance, participating in rituals, providing items needed for compulsions (such as extra soap), modifying schedules, and shaping the family routine in such a way as to minimize the affected child's distress (Lebowitz, Panza, Su, & Bloch, 2012; Storch et al., 2007). For example, parents of a child with contamination fears might engage in ritualized washing of their own hands before handling the child's food. Siblings also report accommodating to the child's anxiety. In one case a brother would regularly lift his older sister in and out of the car because of the fear she had of stepping on the ground in the driveway. This kind of accommodation can cause great distress to the parents or siblings and has been shown to be associated with poorer treatment response as well, with more severe symptoms and greater impairment in the child with OCD.

Generalized Anxiety Disorder

Generalized anxiety disorder (GAD) describes persistent worry, which is difficult to control and is accompanied by tension, restlessness, fatigue, difficulty concentrating, irritability, or sleep disturbance. Although the focus of the worry can vary and may shift or change over time, many children with GAD worry most about their own performance in various domains such as school work or athletic achievement. Other worries that many children report relate to the health of loved ones, being late or making mistakes, or to the family's future, as in worrying about parents getting divorced or about their financial status. Many children with GAD are described by themselves or others as perfectionistic.

Children with GAD typically have somatic symptoms such as complaining about aches or pains, stomach unrest or nausea, or being overly tired. Another feature of GAD is its close association with mood disorders such as depression. In older children generalized anxiety creates a risk for substance abuse, likely as a means of self-medicating the cognitive or physiological symptoms of the chronic stress. The loss of sleep typical of children with GAD can increase the impact of the disorder on both mood and school functioning, making concentration much more difficult. In children whose anxiety focuses on performance or achievement this can create a vicious cycle where the anxiety impairs the ability to perform optimally, which heightens the anxiety about performance. Some children report lying in bed worrying about the sleep they are losing and how it will affect their performance in school the next day, getting more and more worried and accordingly less able to fall asleep.

Parents can become involved in the need to provide reassurance to a child's constant worry, at times needing to respond to many phone calls throughout the day or to answer endless questions prompted by the anxiety. Some children have their parents check and recheck homework assignments with them because of a fear of making a mistake or submitting less than perfect work.

THE GOOD NEWS AND THE BAD NEWS

As discussed earlier in this chapter the various anxiety disorders, despite the differences between them, seem to have more in common with each other than they do distinguishing them. These shared characteristics include two important pieces of information, which we sometimes call the *good news* and the *bad news* of anxiety disorders. The bad news about anxiety is that in most cases, once a disorder has taken hold—in other words is more than a passing worry or a developmentally appropriate fear—the likelihood that the disorder will spontaneously remit is not high. This pattern is due in part to the nature of avoidance, which we discuss more fully in Chapter 5. As children become accustomed to avoiding a given situation, because of anxiety, they experience fewer opportunities to learn that the stimulus is not actually dangerous. In fact, in many cases, if left untreated anxiety disorders will get progressively more severe and lead to more impairment to child and family functioning.

The good news about anxiety disorders, however, is that in the multitude of studies that have been conducted, examining the efficacy of treatment for anxiety disorders, most children have improved dramatically after treatment. Cognitive behavioral therapy (CBT), which is discussed in this book, as well as medication, have been found to be effective ways of treating childhood anxiety. Both of these are now widely considered to be well-supported, evidence-based treatments, which work in most cases.

So what is the conclusion to be drawn from considering both the good and the bad news about anxiety? If left untreated the situation is likely not to improve or even to get worse, but treatment can effectively cure or minimize anxiety disorders, so the obvious conclusion is that treatment is well advised. Unfortunately, due to limitations in access to treatment, dissemination of best practices, and delays in correctly identifying the problem, most children will wait a long time before treatment is attempted.

The Role of Primary Care

One important gateway to treatment that needs to be better utilized is identification and referral by primary care providers. Efforts at various levels, from training of new primary care providers to creating more awareness and influencing policy, are being made to address this need. As Lisa Honigfeld, of the Connecticut-Based Child Health and Development Institute points out, pediatricians, family physicians, nurse practitioners, and other primary care medical providers can play a key role in addressing anxiety. These medical professionals care for children over time, within the context of their families and community environments. Approximately 90% of children and youth visit a primary care provider each year (National Survey of Children's Health, 2007). Such visits are required for school entry and camp and sports participation. These visits, along with sick care visits, present valuable opportunities to identify children who have mental health concerns, a role recognized and endorsed by the American Academy of Pediatrics (Committee on Psychosocial Aspects of Child and Family Health, 2009).

Through open communication and dialogue among parents, primary care providers, and mental health professionals, children at risk for—or already suffering from anxiety disorders—can be identified and offered access to treatment resources. One crucial element is that of screening. When providers of primary care take an active role in screening their patients for symptoms of clinically significant anxiety, the problem can be addressed before some of the more insidious effects of anxiety have taken hold.

Screening can be done at multiple levels, such as inquiring about family history of mental conditions, discussing concerns with parents, asking about anxious or avoidant behavior, and having parents or children (of appropriate age) complete standardized screening tools. Many insurers, including both state and commercial insurance companies, will actually compensate primary care providers for every screening done during a child's well visit. For children over the age of 4, pediatricians can use the Pediatric Symptom Checklist to identify children who may have mental health concerns (Jellinek et al., 1999). Other tools such as the Spence Children's Anxiety Scale are specifically aimed at identifying anxiety-related problems (Spence, Barrett, & Turner, 2003).

Another role in which primary care providers are instrumental is in identifying somatic complaints such as stomachache, disordered sleep, loss of appetite, or headache, which are manifestations of an anxiety disorder. As we discuss more fully in Chapter 6, anxiety has both acute and chronic effects on physiological functioning. In children in partic-ular, who may have difficulty verbalizing their anxiety, somatic com-plaints are a common way of displaying anxiety. In Chapter 14 we discuss the role that anxiety and its somatic component can play in school avoidance and absenteeism.

Although child health-care providers rarely provide psychothera-peutic interventions per se, they can create critical linkages to commu-nity services and can ensure that patients follow through on recommendations for evaluation and counseling. Once children are under the care of mental health professionals for treatment of anxiety, the children's health provider's role is to provide ongoing monitoring of the children's progress toward treatment goals and overall health. This requires regular communication to and from the mental health provider and periodic administration of screening tools and assessment tools.

In the next two chapters we discuss two important facets of childhood anxiety disorders in greater detail. First we look at the relevance of emotion regulation for the development and treatment of anxiety and then at the role of family accommodation in these disorders. The fol-lowing sections of this book focus on treatment of childhood anxiety at the individual and family level. The final section of the book tackles some specific aspects of anxiety such as school phobia and anxiety in adult children and the dependence it can cause.

References

American Psychiatric Association. (2000). *Diagnostic and statistical manual of mental disorders* (4th ed.). Washington, DC: Author.

Angold, A., Messer, S. C., Stangl, D., Farmer, E. M., Costello, E. J., & Burns, B. J. (1998). Perceived parental burden and service use for child and adolescent psychiatric disorders. *American Journal of Public Health, 88*(1), 75–80. doi:10.2105/ajph.88.1.75

Bittner, A. (2007). What do childhood anxiety disorders predict? *Journal of Child Psychology and Psychiatry and Allied Disciplines, 48*(12), 1174.

Brown, L. H., Silvia, P. J., Myin-Germeys, I., & Kwapil, T. R. (2007). When the need to belong goes wrong: The expression of social anhedonia and social anxiety in daily life. [Research Support, Non-U.S. Gov't]. *Psychological Science, 18*(9), 778–782. doi:10.1111/j.1467–9280.2007.01978.x

Committee on Psychosocial Aspects of Child and Family Health (2009). Policy statement – The future of pediatrics: Mental health competencies for pediatric primary care. *Pediatrics, 124*(1), 410–421.

Coplan, R. J., Prakash, K., O'Neil, K., & Armer, M. (2004). Do you "want" to play? Distinguishing between conflicted shyness and social disinterest in early childhood. *Developmental Psychology, 40*(2), 244–258. doi:10.1037/0012–1649.40.2.244

Costello, E. J., Egger, H. L., & Angold, A. (2005). The developmental epidemiology of anxiety disorders: Phenomenology, prevalence, and comorbidity. *Child and Adolescent Psychiatric Clinics of North America, 14*(4), 631–648.

Curry, J. F., March, J. S., & Hervey, A. S. (2004). *Comorbidity of childhood and adolescent anxiety disorders: Prevalence and implications. Phobic and anxiety disorders in children and adolescents: A clinician's guide to effective psychosocial and pharmacological interventions* (pp. 116–140). New York, NY: Oxford University Press.

Jellinek, M. S., Murphy, J. M., Little, M., Pagano, M. E., Comer, D. M., & Kelleher, K. J. (1999). Use of the Pediatric Symptom Checklist to screen for psychosocial problems in pediatric primary care: A national feasibility study. *Archives of Pediatrics and Adolescent Medicine, 153*(3), 254–260.

Keller, M. B., Lavori, P. W., Wunder, J., Beardslee, W. R., Schwartz, C. E., & Roth, J. (1992). Chronic course of anxiety disorders in children and adolescents. *Journal of the American Academy of Child &Adolescent Psychiatry, 31*(4), 595–599. doi:10.1097/00004583–199207000–00003

Kessler, R. C., Berglund, P., Demler, O., Jin, R., Merikangas, K. R., & Walters, E. E. (2005). Lifetime prevalence and age-of-onset distributions of DSM-IV disorders in the national comorbidity survey replication. *Archives of General Psychiatry, 62*(6), 593–602. doi:10.1001/archpsyc.62.6.593

Kessler, R. C., Chiu, W. T., Demler, O., & Walters, E. E. (2005). Prevalence, severity, and comorbidity of 12-month DSM-IV disorders in the national comorbidity survey replication. *Archives of General Psychiatry, 62*(6), 617–627. http://dx.doi.org/10.1001/archpsyc.62.6.617

Klein, D. F. (1993). False suffocation alarms, spontaneous panics, and related conditions. An integrative hypothesis. *Archives of General Psychiatry, 50*(4), 306–317.

Lebowitz, E. R., Panza, K. E., Su, J., & Bloch, M. H. (2012). Family accommodation in obsessive-compulsive disorder. *Expert Review of Neurotherapeutics, 12*(2), 229–238. doi:10.1586/ern.11.200

Lebowitz, E. R., Woolston, J., Bar-Haim, Y., Calvocoressi, L., Dauser, C., Warnick, E., . . . Leckman, J. F. (2012). Family accommodation in pediatric anxiety disorders. *Depression and Anxiety.* doi: 10.1002/da.21998

Merikangas, K. R., He, J.-P., Burstein, M., Swanson, S. A., Avenevoli, S., Cui, L., . . . Swendsen, J. (2010). Lifetime prevalence of mental disorders in U.S. adolescents: Results from the national comorbidity survey replication—Adolescent supplement (NCS-A). *Journal of the American Academy of Child & Adolescent Psychiatry, 49*(10), 980–989. doi:10.1016/j.jaac.2010.05.017

National Survey of Children's Health. (2007). Data Query from the Child and Adolescent Health Measurement Initiative. Retrieved 09/20/2012, from Data Resource Center for Child and Adolescent Health website.

Rapee, R. M., Schniering, C. A., & Hudson, J. L. (2009). Anxiety disorders during childhood and adolescence: Origins and treatment. *Annual Review of Clinical Psychology, 5*(Journal Article), 311–341.

References

Schmidt, N. B., Lerew, D. R., & Trakowski, J. H. (1997). Body vigilance in panic disorder: Evaluating attention to bodily perturbations. *Journal of Consulting and Clinical Psychology, 65*(2), 214–220. doi:10.1037/0022–006x.65.2.214

Spence, S. H., Barrett, P. M., & Turner, C. M. (2003). Psychometric properties of the Spence Children's Anxiety Scale with young adolescents. *Journal of Anxiety Disorders, 17*(6), 605–625.

Storch, E. A., Geffken, G. R., Merlo, L. J., Jacob, M. L., Murphy, T. K., Goodman, W. K., . . . Grabill, K. (2007). Family accommodation in pediatric obsessive-compulsive disorder. *Journal of Clinical Child and Adolescent Psychology, 36*(2), 207–216.

Swedo, S. E., Leckman, J. F., & Rose, N. R. (2012). From research subgroup to clinical syndrome: Modifying the PANDAS criteria to describe PANS (Pediatric Acute-onset Neuropsychiatric Syndrome). *Pediatrics and Therapeutics, 2*(2), doi:10.4172/2161-0665.1000113

Swedo, S. E., Leonard, H. L., Garvey, M., Mittleman, B., Allen, A. J., Perlmutter, S., . . . Dubbert, B. K. (1998). Pediatric autoimmune neuropsychiatric disorders associated with streptococcal infections: Clinical description of the first 50 cases. *American Journal of Psychiatry, 155*(2), 264–271.

Woodward, L. J., & Fergusson, D. M. (2001). Life course outcomes of young people with anxiety disorders in adolescence. *Journal of the American Academy of Child & Adolescent Psychiatry, 40*(9), 1086–1093. doi:10.1097/00004583–200109000–00018

CHAPTER TWO

Anxiety and Emotion Regulation

Self-regulation describes the system by which an individual returns to a state of equilibrium after an event has caused a disruption in some element of functioning. This chapter explores the relationship of childhood anxiety and emotion regulation, including the parental role in fostering more effective regulation by the child.

Key points in this chapter:

- Self-regulation of emotions.
- The relationship of emotion regulation and anxiety.
- The parent-child interaction in the face of regulation challenges.
- Parent guidance as a tool for promoting better emotion regulation.

SELF-REGULATION

Imagine an air conditioner set to 75 degrees. The room it's in feels pleasant—not too cool and not too warm. It feels just right. Then someone opens a window. Outside it's winter and cold air rushes into the room. The thermostat embedded in the air conditioner senses the change and activates heating elements and fans, which start blowing warm air into the room. Soon it's back to 75 and the system settles back into standby mode. If the room were to grow hotter, say if 15 people crowded in for a meeting, the system would respond to that change as well as by activating the cooling mechanism until things were just right again.

This is the essence of regulation: responding to changes in a way that can stabilize the system and restore balance. All through nature and all through life are systems that act to constantly counteract fluctuations and ensure stability. However, not all systems are equally sensitive or equally efficient at regulating the thing they're monitoring.

Sensitivity in regulation describes the degree of change necessary for the regulatory system to become activated. An air conditioner, for instance, might only be activated when the temperature in the room dropped a set number of degrees from the setting. This is necessary because minute fluctuations are always going to be happening, and trying to counteract each and every one would be costly and inefficient. It would require more rapid measurement and a more advanced thermostat. The more sensitive a regulatory system is, the smaller the change necessary to activate it.

Efficiency, on the other hand, can be thought of as measuring the ease with which a regulatory system is able to restore balance and bring itself back to the desired condition after a change has occurred. A really good air conditioner with lots of horsepower and clean filters will be able to easily counteract the open window before the people in the room start feeling overly cold. A less effective system might have to work much harder and for a much longer period of time before things can go back to how they were with the window closed. If the system is too weak it may never be able to maintain the desired temperature until the window is closed, although it will expend great amounts of energy in trying to do so.

All children are faced with the challenge of regulating a great many aspects of their existence, constantly throughout the day. Bodies, like rooms in buildings, need to maintain constant temperature and have sophisticated systems for doing that, including constant monitoring of internal temperature and a slew of practical mechanisms for adjusting the temperature when it is at risk of straying from normal. Even small shifts will activate these mechanisms, making it a highly sensitive system.

Body temperature, however, is only one of many variables that need to be kept relatively constant to maintain successful functioning. In fact, temperature is actually only representative of one kind of variables—the physiological ones that also include, among others, heart rate, respiration, and oxygenation of blood, caloric intake, available fluids, and so forth. But human beings also need to maintain other kinds of variables within healthy limits, such as emotional and cognitive fluctuations.

EMOTIONAL REGULATION

Emotion regulation is the system by which, when something has happened to throw our inner emotional state off kilter, we gradually return to feeling *regular* again and by which "individuals influence which emotions they have, when they have them and how they experience and express those emotions" (Gross, 1998b). It is a vital aspect of emotional life precisely because so many things have the capacity to temporarily affect the way we are feeling. And just like with air conditioners, some people's systems are more efficient than others. Parents of young babies often note the dramatic differences between different children's ability to self-regulate. Most babies wake up at night, especially during the first months of life. But while one child might be easy to soothe with a feeding or even just some rocking, another, once awake, might have great difficulty returning to a state of relaxation. The difference between the children is not necessarily or exclusively related to how stimulated they were when they woke up—it is usually more a factor of how "good they are" at calming back down. Many distraught parents will tell horror stories about their "worst" sleeper, who might need hours of crying and soothing before being relaxed enough to fall back asleep (and allow their exhausted parents to do the same).

The list of things that can affect a child's inner state and require activation of the self-regulatory systems is endless, and includes both good things and not so good things. When something makes a child happy, that feeling is associated with a cascade of physiological and phenomenological alterations that underlie the ensuing feeling of joy. Due to the child's ability to self-regulate, that joy is somewhat short lived and some time later the child is probably feeling "regular" (i.e., self-regulated) again. For most children, even extreme fluctuations of their internal emotional states are quite brief and effectively regulated within a brief period of time.

Even very young babies appear to actively engage in emotional regulation through behaviors such as avoiding stimuli that make them feel unpleasant sensations by averting their gaze or through activating self-soothing behaviors such as sucking when feeling out of sorts. Beyond these somewhat limited tools, infants are dependent on their autonomous systems and on their caretakers to regulate unpleasant states of arousal. Until the ability to self-regulate matures, parents act as a kind of "proxy" for self-regulation, facilitating the child's regulation by such means as soothing touch and speech, rocking, removal of stimuli that are causing arousal, and many others. By the time they reach toddlerhood most children are able to consciously attempt to soothe themselves; for example, by hugging a favorite toy, distracting themselves, or removing themselves from whatever is producing the emotion. Another tool discovered by children around this age is the ability to actively and willingly enlist the help of an adult to achieve emotional regulation. Although this ability is a sign of progress and development, some children will come to rely too exclusively on their ability to mobilize others to help them achieve regulation.

Both biological and environmental factors can impact the effectiveness with which children self-regulate their emotional state (Bronson, 2000; Holodynski & Friedlmeier, 2006). Negative environmental factors include early exposure to prolonged or extreme stressful situations whereas positive ones include sensitive parenting that acknowledges the children's feelings and recognizes their inner states (Fonagy, 2002). An aspect of regulation that exemplifies the importance of biological factors is that of *sensitivity*, which appears to be closely tied to the function of the *locus coeruleus* — a part of the brainstem that produces norepinephrine in response to stressful situations. An overactive locus coeruleus produces the anxiety-related norepinephrine in response to more stimuli, making regulation a much more considerable challenge than it might be for someone with a more "lazy" locus coeruleus.

Emotional Regulation and Anxiety Disorders in Children

The relation between anxiety and self-regulation makes intuitive sense when we recall that the role of anxiety is to aid in avoiding any situation that poses a threat to safety or well-being. When children, because of

26

oversensitivity or ineffective regulation, experience many situations as threatening it is not surprising that their anxiety system will "work overtime" to help in avoiding these situations in the first place. Or, put differently, when a child has greater difficulty regulating negative emotion, the strategy of avoiding potential triggers becomes more appealing. The two concepts are so closely linked that it is impossible to say whether it is being more anxious that places an increased strain on the regulatory system or whether anxiety disorders stem from ineffective regulation. In fact both statements are likely to be true. Either way, bearing the relationship between anxiety and regulation in mind is important in treating anxiety disorders directly, as well as in the context of parent guidance.

Significant amounts of data pointing to the important role of emotion regulation deficits in the formation or maintenance of anxiety disorders have been accumulating for some years. The data come from both neurobiological and behavioral investigations of anxiety. One study (Banks, Eddy, Angstadt, Nathan, & Phan, 2007) underscored the physiological foundation of emotion regulation in anxiety-exposed participants to anxiety-inducing stimuli and then asked them to either remain aware of their feelings but not change them, or to attempt to decrease their anxiety through a process of reappraisal (reinterpreting the content of the picture so that it no longer caused them to feel anxious). Functional magnetic resonance imaging (fMRI) of the subjects' brains during the task revealed that specific areas of the frontal cortex such as the dorsolateral, dorsal medial, anterior cingulate, and orbital were differentially activated based on whether the subject was attempting to engage in emotion regulation of the anxiety. Moreover, the strength of the association between those areas and the amygdala (a component of the brain consistently tied to anxiety) predicted the degree of regulation that the subjects achieved. Amygdala function has also been shown to be more easily activated by anxiety-provoking stimuli in youth suffering from anxiety disorders compared to normal adolescents (Guyer et al., 2008).

Interestingly, there is at least some evidence to show that in much the same way that behavioral avoidance can compound or maintain an anxiety disorder, the attempt to suppress the emotional element of anxiety can also maintain greater degrees of neurophysiological arousal.

27

Individuals who, when exposed to anxiety-inducing stimuli, were asked to mask the anxiety they were feeling and not allow it to show on their face actually demonstrated increases in amygdala activation during the task (Goldin, McRae, Ramel, & Gross, 2008). Similar findings have been reported using peripheral rather than central nervous system measures of anxious arousal (Gross, 1998a). In obsessive-compulsive disorder, in which intrusive thoughts cause negative experiences of anxiety or disgust, attempts at suppressing the thoughts are central to the disorder as children become trapped in a loop that exacerbates their anxiety rather than effectively regulating it (Janeck & Calamari, 1999).

Studies focusing on the behavioral and the cognitive aspects of emotion regulation have also highlighted its role in the context of anxiety disorders. Suveg and Zeman (2004) assessed the emotional regulation of children based on self- and parent report. They found that children who met criteria for an anxiety disorder had more difficulty managing feelings of worry and other negative emotional states, and coped with them less adaptively. They also found that those children reported more intense experiences of worry compared to nonanxious children, furthering the hypothesis that overarousal coupled with less-effective regulation mechanisms may contribute, or perhaps be integral to, anxiety disorders of children.

Environmental and family factors, such as the way parents regulate their own emotions or respond to a child's anxiety can potentially contribute to the link between emotion regulation and anxiety in the child. Hudson and Rapee (2001) observed parents' interactions with their children and found that parents were less able to regulate their own involvement with anxious children, manifesting greater degrees of overinvolvement when interacting with anxious children compared to nonanxious siblings. Additionally, it is likely that children learn self-regulation strategies partially by observing their parents, and that modeling of poor regulation could predispose the child to similar difficulties.

In fact, in our experience and that of others (Zucker & Bradley, 1995), many parents of anxious children do describe their child as *overly sensitive*. Parents usually include in this concept sensitivity to a host of aversive stimuli that trigger the child's negative emotions more easily than they would for the typical child. These might include sensory sensitivity (the child who can't wear any socks but that one pair, or who is always bothered by seams and labels), emotional and relational sensitivity (the kid who is always first to take offense, cries easily, or cannot handle losing and will "melt down" at not winning), food sensitivity ("he only eats three things and he wants them every day"), and many others. However, the studies described earlier highlight the fact that emotion regulation in a child who is anxious is actually an interpersonal construct. Much the same way as anxiety itself is not confined to the child, but rather exists in the interpersonal space between parent and child, regulation, too, is a two-way street. As parents become overwhelmed by their anxious child, they take over more and more of the role of "regulators." Children come to rely on the parents to alleviate the uncomfortable arousal, and the parents become less able to allow children the necessary time to discover their own capacity for self-regulation. Parents of an anxious child face a double challenge—the need to withstand the child's temporary dysregulation and the need to regulate their own anxiety and related emotions. When parents are predisposed to being less effective at regulating their own anxiety, a cycle of dysregulation is created. Parent and child trigger arousal and anxiety in each other, and the child has few opportunities to learn effective regulating strategies.

Parent guidance can help to break this cycle by teaching the parents tools to better regulate themselves, as well as ways in which to model better regulation for their children. The parents learn to allow the child the necessary time to implement those techniques and to withstand the urge to fulfill the regulatory function on the child's behalf by means of avoidance. A helpful way of explaining to parents the state of mind of an anxious child with regard to regulation may be to refer back to the air-conditioner analogy:

A child who tends to be overly anxious is a little like an air conditioner, which is both sensitive and inefficient. It is sensitive in that it is activated by even minor variations in temperature, that another model might not consider significant enough to regulate. It is inefficient in that it takes much longer than others to bring things back to a resting state. The outcome? Being almost always "on"—trying unsuccessfully to maintain regulation. An anxious child can be "activated" by minor stressors that others might "screen out" or ignore, but he also may take a long time to relax after the anxiety is triggered. And the result is persistent and unpleasant arousal that causes ongoing stress.

Another analogy emphasizes the ways in which difficulty in emotion regulation can shape children's views of the world as well as their choices and personality:

> Imagine you are in a minefield. You don't know where the mines are but you know they're all around you, and that a wrong move could cause one to go off. Even if you've never been in a minefield, you can imagine that the way you'd walk would probably be quite different from the way you normally walk. In fact there would probably be two main differences:
>
> First of all you'd probably want to walk as little as possible! After all, if you're standing somewhere right now and all is safe, then any movement can only mean increasing your danger. So you'd probably only walk anywhere if you absolutely had to.
>
> Second, where would you rather step if you really had to go somewhere? Probably you would choose a path that would allow you to only step in places where you'd already stepped before! Definitely best to put your feet only in those spots that were already tested and proven to be safe.

This description captures the essence of the way many anxious children navigate the world, and resonates powerfully with parents time and again. When regulation is a challenge rather than an automatic process, negative events seem much more awful and the risk of triggering them can greatly outweigh the potential for positive experiences. The world seems like a minefield and every negative or unpleasant experience is akin to stepping on a mine. Viewing the world in this way can affect even minor decisions and everyday situations. Consider, for example, how different children approach a new food:

> When a food is unfamiliar there is always the risk that it will be unpleasant. It might have a bitter taste or it may not feel right in my mouth. For most of us such a risk is negligible. After all, if I really don't like it I can always spit it out and not eat it again. But if I'm quite sensitive there are probably many foods that will feel or taste wrong to me; and if regulation is very challenging for me it might take me much longer to

30

recover from the unpleasant experience. In that case I'll probably be willing to lose out on the possibility of discovering a new food that I really like just to avoid the risk of running into a bad experience.

This pattern, too, is familiar to parents of anxious children, who will often report that their child always seems to prefer running the risk of losing out on a good thing rather than taking a chance and exposing themselves to a potentially bad one. When, for one reason or another, children do experience a new stimulus and find it pleasant, they will generally be willing to repeat that particular thing again in the future. However, they might be no more willing to take a new chance on another one. They have found one more safe place to put their feet down in the minefield of life, but have not become convinced that there aren't mines all around. Parents are often frustrated by this because they perceive the child to not be learning from the experience. They may say something like "You see! It pays to take a chance now and then, right?" But the child may still be unprepared to risk potentially dysregulating experiences.

The difficulty parents face in regulating their own anxiety, when confronted with their child's anxiety, can be a powerful factor in bringing about greater degrees of accommodation or negative expressed emotion. Both of these, in turn, have been related to childhood anxiety disorders. In Chapter 9 we discuss family boundaries in the context of childhood anxiety and look at the some of the ways in which a child's anxiety acts to blur the boundaries that would normally separate parent from child. This happens on many levels, but one of them is that of the emotional separation. Anxiety in a child triggers anxiety in parents and can make it hard for parents to distinguish their own feelings from the child's experience. When a child is particularly distressed, or being especially expressive about the anxiety, the parent's emotional self-regulatory system faces a tremendous challenge. In this situation, any father or mother might feel a desperate need to do something, anything, to alleviate the anxiety. The urge to fix the problem can feel acute and a parent may be powerfully motivated to help the child feel better in any way possible. This is compounded by worry about the potentially damaging effect to the child's well-being of experiencing such distress.

In this situation accommodation, discussed from various perspectives throughout this book and described in detail in the next chapter, can seem like the only viable alternative. Providing reassurance, for example, by answering a question that a child is intensely worried about is often all but inevitable. However, more and more research is pointing to the fact that the accommodation actually serves to reinforce the anxiety in the longer term by modeling avoidance. The parent is avoiding anxiety, and the child's belief that this is the only option is strengthened. The parent is also missing an opportunity to model more adaptive self-regulation strategies that the child could potentially learn to adopt.

By refraining from accommodation and engaging in other strategies the parent can send a powerful message to the child about how to deal with anxiety. For example, when a child, faced by a parent's refusal to accommodate asks "Don't you care about how I feel?" a parent might respond by saying "Of course I do, I feel absolutely terrible. But I am telling myself that you will be okay again soon and that you can handle this. That helps me to stay calm," or even "Yes, when I feel like this I think it helps to breathe a little and wait a few minutes before doing anything."

REFERENCES

Banks, S. J., Eddy, K. T., Angstadt, M., Nathan, P. J., & Phan, K. L. (2007). Amygdala–frontal connectivity during emotion regulation. *Social Cognitive and Affective Neuroscience, 2*(4), 303–312. doi:10.1093/scan/nsm029

Bronson, M. (2000). *Self-regulation in early childhood: Nature and nurture.* New York, NY: Guilford Press.

Fonagy, P. (2002). *Affect regulation, mentalization, and the development of the self.* New York, NY: Other Press.

Goldin, P. R., McRae, K., Ramel, W., & Gross, J. J. (2008). The neural bases of emotion regulation: Reappraisal and suppression of negative emotion. *Biological Psychiatry, 63*(6), 577–586. doi:10.1016/j.biopsych.2007.05.031

Gross, J. J. (1998a). Antecedent- and response-focused emotion regulation: Divergent consequences for experience, expression, and physiology. *Journal of Personality and Social Psychology, 74*(1), 224–237.

References

Gross, J. J. (1998b). The emerging field of emotion regulation: An integrative review. *Review of General Psychology, 2*(3), 271–299.

Guyer, A. E., Lau, J. Y., McClure-Tone, E. B., Parrish, J., Shiffrin, N. D., Reynolds, R. C., . . . Nelson, E. E. (2008). Amygdala and ventrolateral prefrontal cortex function during anticipated peer evaluation in pediatric social anxiety. *Archives of General Psychiatry, 65* (11), 1303–1312.

Holodynski, M., & Friedlmeier, W. (2006). *Development of emotions and emotion regulation*. New York, NY: Springer.

Hudson, J. L., & Rapee, R. M. (2001). Parent-child interactions and anxiety disorders: An observational study. *Behaviour Research and Therapy, 39*(12), 1411–1427.

Janeck, A. S., & Calamari, J. E. (1999). Thought suppression in obsessive-compulsive disorder. *Cognitive Therapy and Research, 23*(5), 497–509. doi:10.1023/a:1018720404750

Suveg, C., & Zeman, J. (2004). Emotion regulation in children with anxiety disorders. *Journal of Clinical Child and Adolescent Psychology, 33* (4), 750–759.

Zucker, K. J., & Bradley, S. J. (1995). *Gender identity disorder and psychosexual problems in children and adolescents*. New York, NY: Guilford Press.

CHAPTER THREE

When Anxiety Takes Over — Family Accommodation

A child's anxiety disorder can become a major factor impacting the entire family. Family accommodation describes the changes to family life, aimed at reducing the child's anxiety. Some parents accommodate to the child's anxiety out of a wish to help the child and reduce their distress; in other cases the child may forcibly impose accommodation on the family.

Key points in this chapter:

- Prevalence of family accommodation.
- Significance and implication of family accommodation.
- Some children impose accommodation forcefully through various means such as "emotional blackmail" or disruptive behaviors.

FAMILY ACCOMMODATION

In the previous chapters we discussed the common anxiety disorders of children and the role of emotion regulation for a child's anxiety. However, anxiety in children is best viewed from a perspective that incorporates the whole family rather than only the individual child. In later chapters in this book we discuss this family perspective in detail from both theoretical and practical perspectives and present treatment strategies that stem directly from this view. In the current chapter we focus on one particular aspect of family involvement in a child's anxiety that has important implications for both individual and family based treatment.

Clara was 14½ when she first experienced a panic attack. Her heart pounded and she felt her chest tightening to the point that her breathing was labored. She felt terrified and alone. Although she was in her own backyard she felt unable to call her parents, who were right inside; like someone trapped in a nightmare she tried to call and no sound came out. After she felt better she vowed never to be helpless and alone again. Since that day Clara has avoided going places without her parents. Instead of taking the school bus her parents now drive her to school and pick her up at the end of the day. This is inconvenient as her father likes to leave the house early to avoid rush hour and her mother runs a business from home, but she has refused to go to school unless they promise to drive her both ways. She also is terrified of being the last person awake in the house. She panics if her parents want to go to bed a little early and begs that they give her time to fall asleep first. Clara is constantly searching for signs of another attack. Every hiccup, every heartburn spell impending doom in her mind, and at least once or twice a day she has her mother, who has some medical training, take her blood pressure with a machine they bought expressly for this purpose. Clara is so worried that she asks endless health-related questions and expects her parents to have reassuring answers. On the other hand she challenges their every answer, so that they grow more and more exasperated with her. Her parents feel that they are losing the happy teenager they knew and that her anxiety is taking over their lives, as well as hers.

Family accommodation is a term used to describe the ways in which family members of individuals with anxiety disorders adapt and modify their own behaviors in ways that are aimed at reducing their relative's anxiety. In the context of childhood anxiety, accommodation is most often reported by parents, but siblings, too, are frequently involved in accommodating behaviors. Accommodation typically includes two related categories of changes to parent behavior. These categories are *participation* in behaviors relating to the anxiety, and *modification* of family routines.

Participation in Symptom-Related Behavior

Parents can *participate* in their child's symptom-related behavior in any number of ways. For example, some parents will check all the locks in the house every night together with their child. Others might repeatedly wash their own hands because of a child's fear of dirt and contamination. In fact, most parents of children with compulsive rituals will find themselves engaging in some of the rituals themselves. Another kind of symptom participation entails assisting children in avoiding those situations that make them anxious. For example, when a child is shy, as in the case of social phobia, parents might find themselves speaking instead of the child. Other parents might refrain from going places with a child because they know it will trigger anxiety. For instance, if a child has a fear of heights the family might be extra careful not to drive routes that would mean driving over bridges or near a cliff. Other fears and phobias will dictate other kinds of avoidance and participation.

Another way that parents can participate in children's symptoms is by supplying children with items they need to escape feeling anxious. Some children, for example, will be afraid to leave the house without a water bottle and parents might be extra careful to make sure they always have one on hand. A child with a hand-washing compulsion might go through absurd quantities of soap in short periods of time, and parents will likely find themselves stocking up on what might seem like wholesale supplies for them to wash with. If the parents neglect to keep the house well-stocked, children will have difficulty performing the ritual to alleviate their anxiety. Sometimes participation means simply providing frequent reassurance to a worried child, as in the case of general anxiety disorder and its endless worries. Or perhaps spending nights in a child's bed (or having the child in the parents' bed) because of separation anxiety disorder.

Modification of Family Functioning

Modification describes all the ways in which a family's routines may change in order to prevent one child from experiencing anxiety. When children have separation anxiety, for instance, they might find it difficult or impossible to be home alone after school while the parents are still at work. A typical example of modification would be one parent cutting short the workday to prevent this situation, and help the child avoid feeling anxious. Parent's leisure time can also be affected. Some parents will feel they cannot go out at night and leave an anxious child with a babysitter because of the distress it would cause. As one parent put it:

> By the time we got through the begging, crying, and screaming we were so exhausted we just wanted to go to sleep. There was no point in planning a "date night" for us if it meant dealing with such an ordeal on the way.

Excusing a child from responsibilities such as chores or homework is another common form of modification. In many families of anxious children, leisure activities and vacation plans are modified to avoid anxiety. For example, having a child who is afraid of bees might mean not going to picnics, while one who is afraid of water could spell avoidance of water parks, pools, or beaches. One particularly problematic form of modification involves limiting the entrance of people into the home. When the presence of strangers, guests, or relatives causes the anxious child discomfort, parents may avoid having them, significantly impacting the entire family's social life. Sometimes even siblings are discouraged from having friends over because of a brother or sister who is made uncomfortable by the entrance of any guests.

Prevalence of Family Accommodation

Family accommodation has been studied most thoroughly in the context of one particular anxiety disorder, obsessive-compulsive disorder or OCD. Studies have shown that more than 90% of parents report engaging in at least some forms of accommodation and many do so every day (Lebowitz et al., 2012; Peris, Bergman et al., 2008; E. A. Storch et al., 2007). The Family Accommodation Scale (Calvocoressi et al., 1995) is a measure that is frequently used to assess family accommodation among parents of children suffering from OCD. We recommend assessing family accommodation as part of the evaluation of any child with an anxiety disorder, particularly OCD. Parents are first asked to describe the OCD symptoms that their children demonstrate and are then queried about the extent of their accommodating behaviors, the degree of distress that these cause, and additional consequences of the accommodation or of refusal to accommodate. Another scale, which also contains items designed to probe for accommodating behaviors among parents of children with OCD, is the Parental Attitudes and Behaviors Scale (Peris, Benazon, Langley, Roblek, & Piacentini, 2008).

Accommodation and the Clinical Course of Anxiety

Higher degrees of family accommodation are associated with a number of negative factors in anxiety disorders. Children whose parents report more accommodating behaviors typically have more severe symptoms compared to children whose parents are less accommodating (Caporino et al., 2012; E. Storch et al., 2007). In addition, the degree of impairment caused by the symptoms of anxiety has also been found to be greater when families accommodate more (Storch et al., 2010). It is impossible to say with certainty whether it is the family's accommodating behaviors that are making the symptoms worse, or whether children who have more severe symptoms cause their parents to accommodate more. The studies that have pointed to these links have usually been cross-sectional, relying on information gathered at a single point in time and not allowing for interpretations about causality. The most likely explanation is that both of these things actually do occur. In other words, when parents accommodate more to children's anxiety, their symptoms may increase in severity. They are likely to become more convinced of their inability to function without accommodation and to be less challenged to overcome anxiety. Conversely, children who manifest greater anxiety and more severe symptoms may trigger more accommodation in their surroundings. Whether through sheer number and frequency of symptoms or by appearing more dependent on the accommodation, greater anxiety is likely to produce more accommodation.

Although presumably accommodation usually follows anxiety and not the other way around, it is conceivable that in some cases the accommodation may actually prompt the onset of an anxiety disorder. When might this happen? In cases of children who first display mild or subclinical symptoms of anxiety, which do not yet meet criteria for a full-blown disorder. For example, a child may become increasingly sensitive to dirt without actually suffering from OCD. In fact, it is normal for children, as well as adults, to manifest some degree of anxiety-related symptoms, which, were they to be sufficiently magnified, would constitute a disorder. When this is the case, early overaccommodation may precipitate the symptoms' development into a more clinically significant disorder as the child comes to rely on the mechanism of avoidance rather than coping.

Accommodation and Treatment Outcomes

Family accommodation has also been repeatedly tied to poorer treatment outcomes for children with OCD. In analyzing data collected during the largest and most systematic trial of treatment for childhood OCD (the Pediatric OCD Treatment Study or POTS I), Abbe Garcia (Garcia et al., 2010) found five baseline variables that significantly predicted treatment outcomes. Of these, one was the level of reported family accommodation. Family accommodation was the only family-related variable to predict outcome. In fact, greater family accommodation reported prior to treatment predicted poorer response to treatment across all treatment conditions. In other words, children responded less effectively to cognitive behavioral therapy, medication, or the combination of both treatments when their families engaged in more family accommodation. In another study that compared patients who responded to treatment for OCD to those who did not, the refractory patients were found to be characterized by more family accommodation (Ferrão et al., 2006), although this study focused on adult patients rather than children.

In further support of the relationship between family accommodation and treatment of childhood OCD, parents of children whose treatment was successful reported accommodating less after treatment compared to before (E. Storch et al., 2007; Waters & Barrett, 2000). It seems likely that treatments that focus specifically on reducing accommodation among family members, alongside the more traditional elements of cognitive behavioral therapy such as exposure and response prevention, will fare better than those that do not target accommodation and this hypothesis is already garnering empirical support. For example, in one recently reported study individual child treatment for OCD was augmented by a family-based structured program which was aimed at reducing parental involvement in the disorder. The results showed that reductions in accommodating behavior preceded and predicted improvement in the child's symptoms (Piacentini et al., 2011).

Sibling Accommodation

Siblings of children with anxiety disorders are usually impacted by the anxiety, even when parents are the ones theoretically accommodating to

40

the anxious child's symptoms. For instance, when a family decides to forgo a planned vacation because one child is nervous, the other siblings are almost certainly going to stay home as well. Or, to take a more day-to-day example, some siblings may be asked not to have friends come over to visit when their anxious sibling is home. In cases of obsessive-compulsive disorder the siblings may be seen as a source of contamination and be required to refrain from touching the affected sibling's things or even from sitting on particular chairs or sofas. In other examples, the entire family may need to limit what they watch on television because particular content triggers anxiety or some words may become taboo, forbidden from being spoken in the home because of the fear they cause.

Data on sibling accommodation is relatively scarce; however, the little that is known points to it being both prevalent and important. In one study that assessed sibling accommodation before and after treatment for OCD, the investigators used a version of the Family Accommodation Scale that had been adapted for sibling use. They reported that accommodation by siblings was prevalent before treatment and significantly reduced after treatment compared to patients in a wait-list control group (Barrett, Healy-Farrell, & March, 2004).

ACCOMMODATION ACROSS ANXIETY DISORDERS

Despite the clear potential of all anxiety disorders to impact parents and siblings in many of the same ways that OCD can, there has been surprisingly little attention devoted to the construct in other anxiety disorders. To our knowledge a recent study conducted by our group at the Yale Child Study Center, in collaboration with additional centers, was the first to systematically address this issue (Lebowitz, Woolston, et al., 2012). The potential of a child's anxiety to impact the family has long been recognized and a number of frameworks, including Family Systems Theory, have been used to describe this. However, there has been no other report of a systematic attempt to document the phenomenon, measure its frequency or severity, or relate it to severity of symptoms or to treatment outcomes.

In our study of family accommodation across childhood anxiety disorders, parents of more than 70 children suffering from a range of anxiety disorders including separation anxiety, generalized anxiety, social phobia, and specific phobias reported on their experiences. The parents completed the Family Accommodation Scale—Anxiety (FASA), which was adapted to better relate to the broader spectrum of children's anxious symptoms.

The results of this study confirmed our hypothesis that family accommodation, far from being specific to OCD, was prevalent across all anxiety disorders. More than 90% of parents interviewed reported engaging in accommodating behaviors relating to their child's anxiety. Almost all parents reported participating in symptoms-related behaviors and most described modification to the family's schedules resulting from the need to adjust to the child's anxiety. Most parents also described experiencing distress as a result of the accommodation as well as negative consequences, such as temporary exacerbation of symptoms or aggressive behavior on the part of the child, if they refused to accommodate.

Imposed Accommodation—Coercive Behaviors in Childhood OCD

> There were whole nights when she was awake until three or four in the morning because of the time it would take her to clean a dish. She would wash it over and over again with soap and she forced me to stay with her until morning. If at three in the morning I tried to say "Sweetie, I really need to sleep" she would throw herself on the floor screaming "You don't love me, you don't care about me, you hate me."

Most of the research into family accommodation focuses on asking the parents and relatives of people with OCD whether and how they accommodate to their child's disorder. However, as anxiety and accommodation, by their very nature, are interpersonal phenomena in that it is always one person accommodating to the anxiety of another individual, this can only capture part of the picture. Some aspects of the interaction are difficult to study in this way. One question that was difficult to answer using a tool like the Family Accommodation Scale is how children might get their parents to accommodate. How might accommodation be imposed on parents who would not otherwise be willing to accommodate the symptoms? In our experience, many parents react to the descriptions of accommodation, which we commonly see, with remarks such as "Well, I would never agree to that!" So how do so many parents go from "Absolutely not" to constant accommodation? What do anxious children have at their disposal to impose accommodation on the family? Although the Family Accommodation Scale does ask parents to report on the distress caused by the accommodation and on the severity of negative outcomes of refusing to accommodate, it cannot provide a picture of those outcomes.

We describe *coercive behaviors* in the context of anxiety or obsessive-compulsive disorders as behaviors on the part of the child that are directed toward ensuring that parents continue to accommodate, even against their will. When parents are asked about such behaviors the reports can be quite remarkable. A qualitative study of coercive behaviors, based on in-depth interviews with parents, resulted in a portrayal of almost tyrannical control on the part of some children (Lebowitz, Vitulano, & Omer, 2011). Parents described forceful and even physically violent behaviors that were triggered by refusal to accommodate. Others described the use of various kinds of emotional blackmail such as the accusation that "You don't love me" or threats of self-injury and suicide. The accommodations imposed in these ways included rules the parents were forced to abide by, prohibitions against various behaviors that caused discomfort, and compulsive behaviors of the child that negatively impacted the environment. In one case a child who feared becoming contaminated through contact with her younger sister forbade the sister to touch any of her things, insisted that her mother wash all their clothes separately, and eventually prohibited the sister from even crossing her field of vision! In another case a child who was afraid of stepping on the floor of the house because of a fear of bugs insisted that his parents wheel him around the house on a wheelchair and even lift him over the toilet when he needed to use the bathroom.

To evaluate the frequency of such situations and the degree to which others in the field encountered them, we conducted an international survey among experts in childhood OCD. Responders to the survey included more than 100 experts from 27 different countries around the globe. Ninety-nine percent of the experts who participated in the survey reported seeing similar coercive behaviors in the course of their work. The majority of experts reported that the imposed accommodation was typical of at least one quarter of all cases of pediatric OCD. From other items on the survey we learned that mothers were, perhaps predictably, the most frequent targets of the coercive behaviors, in the responders' experience. Fully 99% of responders identified mothers as primary targets of the behaviors. Another interesting finding was that the majority of participants felt that the coercive behaviors were not the outcome of classical comorbidity between OCD and a disruptive behavior disorder such as oppositional-defiant disorder or conduct disorder. In other words, rather than seeing the coercive children as having two disorders, the participants felt that the coercive behaviors were better explained as part of the obsessive-compulsive disorder itself. Relatedly, the majority also indicated that when the OCD symptoms abated, the coercive-disruptive behaviors generally ceased as well, and were not simply transferred in equal intensity to a new domain.

One outcome of the study of coercive behaviors in the context of childhood OCD was the ability to formulate a more structured checklist that could serve as a tool for identifying and assessing such situations in other families. Based on the results of the qualitative study we devised a checklist that includes 18 items intended to probe the existence and severity of coercive behaviors manifested by some children and adolescents with OCD (Lebowitz et al., 2011). The full scale is included as an appendix at the end of this book.

Research using the CD-POC seems to confirm the idea that the coercive behaviors are indeed secondary to the OCD rather than a manifestation of a comorbid disruptive behavior disorder. This supports the notion of a separate and distinct pattern of disruptive behavior typical of some children with obsessive-compulsive disorder. In fact, when screened with a more classical checklist such as the Child Behavior Checklist, even very coercive behaviors may not be easily detected among children with OCD.

Understanding Coercive Behaviors

Although avoidance is the primary product of anxiety, another outcome of feeling overly anxious is a heightened need for control. Without control children feel powerless against the fears that trouble them. A story told by the father of a young girl with an anxiety disorder exemplifies this point:

> On our last family vacation we visited a small and picturesque village in Europe. Strolling through the narrow alleys, and between the stores and

stands, we lost all track of time. We lost ourselves in the crowded winding streets, and had a wonderful time. Only Michelle, our 10-year-old daughter, didn't seem to enjoy herself at all. She was nervous, and kept bothering us with questions: "What! Lost ourselves? We're lost?!"; "When will we go back to the hotel?"; "How are we going to find the car?"; "Let's ask for help!" "There, I see a policeman, should we call him? Will he know English?"

The ability to wander aimlessly without a clear sense of time or location requires a temporary relinquishment of the usual need for control. Although under normal circumstances getting lost can be an unpleasant experience, on vacation when we are set free from our routine obligations, we can actually enjoy being flexible and letting go of our usual need to be the masters of every situation. However, this flexibility relies on a basic underlying sense that "everything is okay." It's impossible to enjoy being lost, without the knowledge that it's only a temporary situation, which one can instantly change should the need arise. It is only the basic feeling of security, and the relief of letting go of responsibility, which turns relinquishing control, or *letting go*, from a threatening experience into a pleasant one. For 10-year-old Michelle, who did not feel secure enough in the unfamiliar surroundings, losing control was a horrible experience. Although other family members enjoyed wandering aimlessly from alley to alley, Michelle felt that she, her parents, and her sisters were lost in a frightening maze. Her experience was more like a terrifying fairy tale, such as *Hansel and Gretel*, than like her family's pleasant afternoon. Everyone else's lack of concern only made her anxiety worse. She felt like she was the only responsible one in the whole family!

Feeling in control is always to some extent an illusion, given the unpredictable nature of the world. However, it is that feeling that allows one to navigate reality without being constantly assailed by fear. This is precisely the reason that anxious, and particularly obsessive children (Moulding & Kyrios, 2006) with heightened sensitivity to dangers, real or imagined, may strive for greater control and will often attempt to attain it at almost all costs. Supporting an anxious child requires acknowledging this need and honoring his or her feelings. Without this it is an uphill battle to teach the child to relinquish control or better regulate the anxiety.

In some cases, such as the coercive-disruptive behaviors described earlier, the need for control can gradually erode the personal boundaries and create a sense of almost tyrannical domination. Questions aimed at increasing predictability such as "Where are you going?" or "When will you be back" can turn into extreme or forcefully imposed demands to know every parental movement or to refrain from going out at all. As a child comes to rely more and more fully on her ability to attain a sense of control by controlling others, the result can be extremely disruptive.

In the case of OCD, the persistent doubt that is one of the hallmarks of the disorder can translate into the need for reassurance at a variety of levels. In some cases the doubt may center on the relationship itself, such as when a child experiences doubt about being loved and needs constant proof and reassurance of his parents' feelings. The result is a trap that both parent and child fall into as parents try to reassure and the child never achieves more than transient feelings of confidence.

One of the risks associated with the ability to impose accommodation on the family is the risk for lessened willingness to engage with the world outside of the home. No child is able to control the whole world including school and other out-of-home environments. The result is that for some children the world can become divided into two spheres: the home where anxiety is not challenged but rather accommodated, and the rest of the world where many triggers for anxiety exist and cannot be controlled. It is clear that given this view of things many children may opt to spend as much time as possible inside the home. This presents a clear danger for their ability to function outside. Studies have pointed to a role for family accommodation in mediating the relationship between severity of symptoms and the degree of functional impairment they cause to the child. Although the exact mechanisms of this mediating role need to be better researched, it is likely that the mechanism we have described is an important part. In other words, children who can control their home environment are faced with an unhealthy choice: stay home (with less-adaptive functioning) and do not face the anxiety, or engage with the world but relinquish control. The unfortunate fact is that this is not really a choice but a trap that many children are unable to overcome independently. For the child whose family does not accommodate, on the other hand, there is not this kind of refuge. This child must constantly find other ways to overcome anxiety, and the motivation to stay home or to self-isolate from other parts of the world is likely much smaller.

REFERENCES

Barrett, P., Healy-Farrell, L., & March, J. S. (2004). Cognitive-behavioral family treatment of childhood obsessive-compulsive disorder: A controlled trial. *Journal of the American Academy of Child & Adolescent Psychiatry, 43*(1), 46–62.

Calvocoressi, L., Lewis, B., Harris, M., Trufan, S. J., Goodman, W. K., McDougle, C. J., & Price, L. H. (1995). Family accommodation in obsessive-compulsive disorder. *American Journal of Psychiatry, 152*(3), 441–443.

Caporino, N., Morgan, J., Beckstead, J., Phares, V., Murphy, T., & Storch, E. (2012). A structural equation analysis of family accommodation in pediatric obsessive-compulsive disorder. *Journal of Abnormal Child Psychology, 40*(1), 133–143.

Ferrão, Y., Shavitt, R., Bedin, N., de Mathis, M., Carlos Lopes, A., Fontenelle, L., . . . Miguel, E. C. (2006). Clinical features associated to refractory obsessive-compulsive disorder. *Journal of Affective Disorders, 94*(1–3), 199–209.

Garcia, A., Sapyta, J., Moore, P., Freeman, J., Franklin, M., March, J., & Foa, E. B. (2010). Predictors and moderators of treatment outcome in the pediatric obsessive compulsive treatment study (POTS I). *Journal of the American Academy of Child & Adolescent Psychiatry, 49*(10), 1024–1033.

Lebowitz, E. R., Omer, H., & Leckman, J. F. (2011). Coercive and disruptive behaviors in pediatric obsessive–compulsive disorder. *Depression and Anxiety, 28*(10), 899–905.

Lebowitz, E. R., Panza, K. E., Su, J., & Bloch, M. H. (2012). Family accommodation in obsessive–compulsive disorder. *Expert Review of Neurotherapeutics, 12*(2), 229–238.

Lebowitz, E. R., Vitulano, L. A., & Omer, H. (2011). Coercive and disruptive behaviors in pediatric obsessive compulsive disorder: A qualitative analysis. *Psychiatry, 74*(4).

Lebowitz, E. R., Woolston, J., Bar-Haim, Y., Calvocoressi, L., Dauser, C., Warnick, E., . . . Leckman, J. F. (2012). Family accommodation in pediatric anxiety disorders. *Depression and Anxiety*. doi: 10.1002/da.21998

Moulding, R., & Kyrios, M. (2006). Anxiety disorders and control related beliefs: The exemplar of obsessive-compulsive disorder (OCD). *Clinical Psychology Review, 26*(5), 573–583.

Peris, T. S., Benazon, N., Langley, A., Roblek, T., & Piacentini, J. (2008). Parental attitudes, beliefs, and responses to childhood obsessive compulsive disorder: The parental attitudes and behaviors scale. [Peer Reviewed]. *Child & Family Behavior Therapy, 30*(3), 199–214.

Peris, T. S., Bergman, R. L., Langley, A., Chang, S., McCracken, J. T., & Piacentini, J. (2008). Correlates of accommodation of pediatric obsessive-compulsive disorder: Parent, child, and family characteristics. *Journal of the American Academy of Child & Adolescent Psychiatry, 47* (10), 1173–1181.

Piacentini, J., Bergman, R. L., Chang, S., Langley, A., Peris, T., Wood, J., & McCracken, J. (2011). Controlled comparison of family cognitive behavioral therapy and psychoeducation/relaxation training for child obsessive-compulsive disorder. *Journal of the American Academy of Child & Adolescent Psychiatry, 50*(11), 1149–1161.

Storch, E., Geffken, G., Merlo, L., Mann, G., Duke, D., Munson, M., . . . Goodman, W. K. (2007). Family-based cognitive-behavioral therapy for pediatric obsessive-compulsive disorder: Comparison of intensive and weekly approaches. *Journal of the American Academy of Child & Adolescent Psychiatry, 46*(4), 469–478.

Storch, E., Larson, M., Muroff, J., Caporino, N., Geller, D., Reid, J., . . . Murphy, T. K. (2010). Predictors of functional impairment in pediatric obsessive-compulsive disorder. *Journal of Anxiety Disorders, 24*(2), 275–283.

Storch, E. A., Geffken, G. R., Merlo, L. J., Jacob, M. L., Murphy, T. K., Goodman, W. K., . . . Grabill, K. (2007). Family accommodation in pediatric obsessive-compulsive disorder. *Journal of Clinical Child and Adolescent Psychology, 36*(2), 207–216.

Waters, T. L., & Barrett, P. M. (2000). The role of the family in childhood obsessive-compulsive disorder. *Clinical Child and Family Psychology Review, 3*(3), 173–184.

PART TWO

Working with the Anxious Child

The following four chapters describe various components of anxiety and some of the tools for treating anxious children, as well as for providing guidance to their parents. In these chapters we have attempted to provide a broad view of anxiety and its treatment, suitable for working with a wide variety of anxiety disorders, and a wide variety of children. We include in each chapter sections on parent guidance relating to the techniques and strategies described. In a later section we present a manual for working with the parents of those children who are not yet able or willing to participate themselves in treatment.

One of the most frustrating and discouraging experiences a child can have in therapy is that of not being a "good enough patient." When a child is actively participating in treatment and is motivated to overcome anxiety, the feeling that you're letting everyone down—your parents, your therapist, yourself—can be awful. Unfortunately that is the experience that some children will have and ironically it is one of the best features of modern psychotherapy that will cause it.

Where in the past therapy was a flexible, relatively unstructured and open-ended process, today's therapists are increasingly reliant on manuals and "cookbooks" to tell them what to do in treatment. This tendency brings with it a great many advantages. It allows us to make comparisons of different therapeutic approaches because we can assume that the specific clinicians doing the work are less of an influence than the strategy guiding them and it allows therapists to base their work on well-established guidelines that have been shown to be successful for others. It also allows providers such as insurance carriers to make reasonable decisions about what treatments are reliably going to serve the patients and within what time frame.

Although the authors of this book have done (and continue to do) their share in promoting this structured approach to treatment and although this book attempts to present clinicians with useful tools and suggestions on how to implement therapy for anxiety (and even includes an actual manual for working with parents of noncollaborative children), we recognize that the drive toward structured treatment and manualized interventions also carries with it some serious risks. When therapists begin to pay more attention to a manual than to their patient, they are heading for trouble.

With this in mind we have chosen to present the following chapters on working directly with children less as a manual and more as a toolbox. Every child should be offered as many of the tools as possible but no child will take equally well to all of them. Just as some people are always going to come back to that one thing that works best for them, each child will probably find some, but not all, of the tools to be particularly well suited to his or her personality or frame of mind. We recommend encouraging all children to experiment with as many of the tools as possible, as in our experience even the patients themselves are often not that good a guesser in trying to predict what will be helpful to them. But making clear that these are "experiments" aimed at discovering the best approaches for them rather than assignments to be passed or failed can eliminate much of the potential frustration when something just doesn't click.

The diverse nature of the anxious response, including cognitive, emotional, physiological, and behavioral components underscores the futility of insisting that children follow a rigidly prescribed program rather than adapting treatment to their skills and style. It confirms the wisdom of introducing as many techniques as possible but acknowledging the children's ability to choose those that speak most to them. This is what the toolbox metaphor is all about. Allowing children to become familiar with a variety of skills and developing proficiency in those that best suit their particular characteristics.

Why then do we follow this less-structured section with a manual for working with children who are not ready to collaborate with treatment for their anxiety? The answer is that this population of children, although very large, have not received the attention and consideration that have been focused on more collaborative children. Although many books and manuals exist for treating children who are willing to participate in therapy, no such materials exist to guide the therapist in helping the child who does not want help. This is no surprise. However, in the absence of any structured treatment protocols we have developed our approach into a full-fledged manual, hoping that this will help other clinicians and researchers to adopt the techniques we describe. This section on treating anxious children is therefore followed by a section on working exclusively with parents. We first discuss the theoretical basis for the parent-based model and then the manual for a novel parent-based treatment called the *SPACE Program*. Early results from clinical trials of this treatment are encouraging, pointing to the possibility of being able to help children who would otherwise be largely considered outside of the domain of behavioral therapy. It is also our hope that by providing the SPACE Program manual we will encourage others in the field to join with us in subjecting this treatment to the rigors of scientific investigation.

CHAPTER FOUR

Cognitive Tools for Treating Anxiety

Anxiety affects the thought processes in powerful ways, causing children to misinterpret situations, exaggerate their assessments of risk, and focus narrowly on perceived danger. However, cognitions also provide an important key to overcoming anxiety by changing maladaptive thought patterns and learning cognitive skills to battle anxiety.

Key points in this chapter:

- Anxiety can cause significant shifts to the cognitive patterns of children.
- Cognitive restructuring can be used to identify and modify anxiety-driven cognitions.
- The imagination can be used to change the way thoughts drive avoidant behavior.
- Parents can play an important role by changing their own cognitions about the child's anxiety and modeling adaptive cognitive patterns.

THE COGNITIVE ELEMENT OF ANXIETY

Anxiety always has a cognitive element to it. In fact, imagining an anxiety system that did not have an effect on thought patterns seems absurd. Imagine being in real danger, your heart racing, your palms sweating—and not having any thoughts to go along with it, or being completely carefree in mind. This would be unhelpful in the extreme as it would not allow you to direct that anxious energy toward achieving safety or confronting the danger. Even in the case of panic attacks that occur without a clear trigger, the person experiencing the attack will have very different thoughts than at other times. We discuss some of the most important ways in which anxiety affects cognitions, and then discuss tools for addressing the cognitive element of anxiety. We discuss the ways in which parents' cognitions are equally relevant to a child's anxiety and how the strategies presented can be implemented by parents or promoted in the home.

Prevalence of Anxious Thoughts and Misinterpretation of Cues

The basic cognitive component of anxiety is thinking anxious thoughts. These may be worrisome thoughts about things that could go wrong in life like getting sick or not doing well in school; they may be thoughts about specific feared events like a home invasion or getting laughed at; they may be intrusive obsessive thoughts that recur uncontrollably or they may be thoughts about the anxiety itself, such as the idea that it will never go away or will "ruin my life." Anxious children consistently report having frequent thoughts about negative things (Beck, Emery, & Greenberg, 2005) and feeling distressed by these thoughts.

The anxious cognitions of fearful children form both a general negative view of the world, a kind of fearful lens, through which many different experiences and situations are evaluated, as well as more specific biases in attending to stimuli and interpreting them. The general perspective is often termed a *schema* (Beck, 2008). An example of an anxiety-related schema is "People are hostile" or "I am vulnerable." Seeing the world through such a lens will predispose the individual to experience heightened anxiety across many different situations and scenarios (Teachman, 2005). A child who believes that people are hostile will feel anxious about meeting new people because of a fear of being hurt by them. Similarly the schema "I am vulnerable" will cause the child to fear a broad range of situations in which harm is a possibility. A child who holds the opposite schema (i.e., "I am strong and resilient" or "Things usually go my way") will be accordingly less likely to experience trepidation in uncertain circumstances.

Anxiety primes the individual to recognize danger even when none seems to be apparent. Cues and stimuli that most children would consider neutral or even pleasant may be feared or seen as threatening, and in ambiguous situations an anxious person is likely to favor a more negative interpretation than someone less anxious (Lira Yoon & Zinbarg, 2007; MacLeod & Cohen, 1993). Even impressions that are so fleeting that they cannot be consciously registered or processed by the mind can trigger heightened anxiety when a child is keenly attuned to potential danger.

Possessing an anxious schema about the world shapes not only the interpretation of events but also the attention that is paid to various aspects of any situation (Logan & Goetsch, 1993) and the kind of details that the person remembers later (Moradi, Taghavi, Neshat-Doost, Yule, & Dalgleish, 2000; Russo et al., 2006). Fearful children who hear from a friend about their house being burglarized, for example, are likely to focus intently on that information while discarding information about all the children whose houses were not broken into, as well as the fact that their own house was not. When asked to recall the details of a story, anxious children are more likely to recall details that heighten anxiety than those that would potentially serve to mitigate it. Anxious individuals also take longer to disengage from an anxiety-related stimulus and refocus on other aspects of the situation than those who are more anxious (Fox, Russo, Bowles, & Dutton, 2001).

Tunnel Vision

Imagine you're walking home and crossing a busy street after a long day. All kinds of things are going through your mind: how hungry you are; what you still need to get done today; that new book you want to read; a friend you saw earlier; **that huge truck about to run you over**; where you left your phone . . . .

This is preposterous! If people are about to get hit by a truck they don't wonder where they left their phone. There is little point in focusing on anything else until the immediate danger has been avoided. For this reason, when children are anxious it is often hard to get them to focus on anything apart from their anxiety. This kind of tunnel vision can be wearying for both child and parent when the anxiety is chronic and ongoing. It seems as if all the child wants to talk about is fears and this can soon take a toll on the entire family. Helping both parent and child to understand why this pattern actually makes sense is a step toward alleviating some of that anxiety, even before taking active steps to change the maladaptive cognitive patterns.

Another way to picture the effect that anxiety can have on a child's ability to concentrate on unrelated tasks is to consider how threats tend to grab our attention:

> Imagine yourself sitting in a classroom completing a test the teacher has just handed out. You start to work on answering the questions when you notice thick black smoke billowing into the room from under the door and between the vents. It seems as though you are the only one to notice the smoke and you are instructed to ignore it and just concentrate on the test. How successful would you be on that test? Would you be able to ignore the clear danger signal and focus on the test questions? Could you "tune out" the smoke and choose not to think about it?

This example may help to illustrate the frustration that many children will feel when given the unhelpful, but inevitable advice to "not think about it." It is really not possible to choose not to think about a worrying thought. All too often a child's ability to focus successfully on any cognitive task will suffer significantly because of the intrusion of anxious cognitions.

Although studying attentional disengagement is difficult, a considerable body of research has utilized experimental designs to probe the tendency of anxious individuals to remain focused on negative stimuli longer than less anxious people. In one design a person facing a computer screen is presented with various neutral or fearful faces on either side of the screen, and then required to respond to a cue that appears on one side of the screen. Results have repeatedly shown that responding to cues that appear further from the fearful face takes longer for anxious, compared to nonanxious individuals (Amir, Elias, Klumpp, & Przeworski, 2003; Roy et al., 2008). This has also been supported by the finding that the anxiety provoking cues generated greater fear-typical brain activation associated with the lower response time (Bar-Haim, Lamy, & Glickman, 2005; Monk et al., 2006).

Overestimating Risks

Anxious children also tend to exaggerate the likelihood that negative events will occur. This tendency is another example of how the adaptive survival-oriented role of anxiety can be "hijacked" when a child has an anxiety disorder (Maner & Schmidt, 2006). By assuming the worst, one can be better prepared for it, and when children are overly anxious, seeing prospective undesirable events as more likely to occur allows children to feel that they are preparing for those events rather than complacently supposing that all will be well. Like all symptoms of anxiety disorders, when the anxiety takes on a negative role impeding a child's ability to engage in appropriate behaviors, the persistent sense of impending catastrophe can have a detrimental effect on well-being.

One way in which anxiety affects risk appraisal is through emotion-based information processing and decision making (Angie, Connelly, Waples, & Kligyte, 2011; Loewenstein, Hsee, Weber, & Welch, 2001). When faced with uncertainty about how to interpret a given situation or how to act during it, individuals rely partly on their own inner emotional state as a kind of built-in compass. When feeling anxious they are more likely to perceive the current event or stimulus as more dangerous than at other, more emotionally relaxed times. In essence, children are using their own level of anxiety to gauge actual risk. Children ask themselves "How anxious do I feel?" and if the answer is "Very" they assume that risk must be imminent. This kind of processing is unhelpful when a disorder is causing the child to feel more anxious than necessary.

Cognitive Avoidance

In Chapter 5 we explore the primary behavioral outcome of anxiety, *avoidance*. However, avoidance does not only happen in actual or physical behavior, as when a child with a fear of heights refuses to look out a window. It can also happen at the cognitive level—when a child attempts to block thoughts that cause anxiety. Unfortunately, in most cases not only is cognitive avoidance not successful, but paradoxically it actually causes exacerbation of the anxious ideation. An example is children who imagine themselves being kidnapped and feel afraid as a consequence. Children may say to themselves "I must not think that thought" or "I want never to think that again." By doing so they are almost certainly ensuring that the thought will reappear within a short amount of time, at which point it will arouse an even more negative response. Now the children are not only afraid of the actual thought (being kidnapped), they are also likely feeling frustrated at their own inability to block the thought and to prevent its recurrence.

Children, who have a natural tendency to magical thinking (Rees, Draper, & Davis, 2010) and an egocentric view of the world, (Libby, Reynolds, Derisley, & Clark, 2004) are particularly susceptible to a certain kind of negative reaction to anxious thoughts. They often come to believe that the very act of thinking a certain thing actually increases the likelihood of the imagined outcome happening in real life. When this happens, the need to avoid certain thoughts becomes ever more important, even as the attempts to do so remain completely futile. One additional emotionally-laden reason that children will feel the need to avoid even thinking about negative events is that these can cause them to feel guilty. As though by imagining something bad happening they are expressing a wish for it to happen or are guilty of some other sin. This, as well as other aspects of cognitive avoidance, is particularly typical of children with obsessive-compulsive disorder, which is usually characterized by intrusive distressing thoughts and by ineffective attempts to block them.

Yet another form of cognitive avoidance happens when children are unwilling to voice clearly, to themselves or to others, just what it is that they fear. Children, as well as adults, will often stop short of explicitly stating their most frightening thoughts, preferring to replace them with milder or euphemistic alternatives. For example, children who are afraid to stay home alone, when asked what it is that they think could happen if they were to do so, may respond with a very general "something bad could happen to them," meaning their parents. Although it may appear as though the child has answered the question, this is actually usually an example of avoidance rather than a clarification. When pressed to be more specific, children will often state that they do not have any answer or are not sure themselves of what the potentially bad thing is. It has been our experience that although this is true in some cases, for many children explicating their fear is an exposure in itself and one that they prefer to avoid. However, maintaining such avoidance allows the fears to retain a certain power. The sense that a thought is too terrible to even be spoken about adds to its aura of terror, whereas the thought that has been clearly stated loses some of its mystique.

One way to explain this to children draws on an example familiar to many of them: Lord Voldemort in the Harry Potter series:

> Think about what Voldemort is called by almost everyone in the Harry Potter books: "He who must not be named." Why do you think he wants to be called that instead of by his name? Because Voldemort stays powerful by making everyone afraid of him! He know that if people are so afraid they cannot even say his name they will definitely be too afraid to challenge him! Who is the only person who calls him by his name? Harry! He's the only one who refuses to be afraid and is willing to challenge him. When we are so afraid of our thoughts that we cannot even speak them we are also going to be afraid to challenge them.

Another helpful strategy in such cases can be to ask the child about negative events that could happen to *other* children in a similar situation. Doing so can reduce some of the fear triggered by stating the thought, or encourage children to voice their fears for the first time even to themselves. Once the cognitions have been spoken about clearly, it is usually easy to bring the conversation back to the child himself and base it on what he or she has said.

Next are some helpful tools that parents and children can learn to combat the negative cognitive effects of anxiety.

Cognitive Restructuring: Challenging the Anxious Thoughts

This technique can be taught to both children and adults and, like most skills, is better practiced in a nonanxiety-provoking situation first, until the necessary skill is achieved to start implementing it in "real-life" events. Cognitive restructuring refers to the practice of identifying the anxious thoughts that are making a child fearful and then challenging those thoughts and replacing them with more realistic estimations and assessments.

A typical example might be:

THERAPIST: Tell me what you're nervous about.

PATIENT: I'm afraid my mom will get in an accident while I'm out of the house.

THERAPIST: I see, that does sound scary. Do you think it's likely that that will actually happen?

PATIENT: It could happen!

THERAPIST: Yes, true . . . it could, but has your mother been driving for a while now?

PATIENT: Yes, for 30 years.

THERAPIST: And how many serious accidents has she had?

PATIENT: I don't know, none I think.

THERAPIST: Oh! It sounds like she must have driven a lot in that time right?

PATIENT: I guess . . . she drives every day.

THERAPIST: Right, so she's driven thousands and thousands of times and never had an accident?

PATIENT: Right.

THERAPIST: So you'd agree that the chances of her having an accident this time are pretty slim aren't they?

PATIENT: Yes, pretty slim.

In this example the therapist is leading the patient to recognize the overestimation of threat that has been occurring by demonstrating the rarity of the dreaded event. The following stages would involve children learning to replace the negative ideation with more realistic ones on their own. By doing so, not only is the anxiety being challenged but a distance is being created separating the child from anxiety and placing the thoughts in the position of an external disturbance to be addressed rather than an opinion the child identifies with.

Another example of cognitive restructuring (this time with a socially anxious young man) might be:

THERAPIST: Tell me about what happened in the lunch room at school the other day.

PATIENT: I was sitting at my table, with some other kids when I saw two guys from my class whispering to each other and sort of giggling.

THERAPIST: And what went through your mind? What did that make you think?

PATIENT: I thought "They're laughing at me; I must look funny or they just think I'm weird."

THERAPIST: And how did that make you feel? What happened next?

PATIENT: I wanted to get out of there. It felt bad and I could feel my cheeks burning. I just dumped what was left on my tray in the garbage and went back to the classroom. I haven't been back in the lunchroom since then. I just can't eat there.

THERAPIST: What have you been doing for lunch?

PATIENT: I got permission to eat in my class. I bring a sandwich and eat at my desk.

THERAPIST: So, thinking they were laughing at you made you feel bad, and you've been avoiding the possibility that you'll feel like that again?

PATIENT: Right. What's the point of going to the lunchroom if I can't eat there?

THERAPIST: Would it have felt different if they were laughing at something else; if they weren't laughing at you at all?

PATIENT: Well, sure. If I knew they were not laughing at me I wouldn't care that they were giggling like that. But I'm pretty sure they were.

THERAPIST: Okay, I understand that. Hypothetically though, can you think of anything else they *might* have been laughing at? Anything at all?

PATIENT: I guess so. They could be remembering something that happened earlier that day?

THERAPIST: Great. That's just what I mean! What other things *might* they have been laughing at?

PATIENT: I guess they might be telling a joke.

THERAPIST: Yes.

PATIENT: Maybe planning something funny? But they really looked like they were laughing at someone.

THERAPIST: Okay. And if they were in fact laughing at someone, is it at all possible that they just might have been' laughing at someone other than you?

PATIENT: Well, sure that's possible. I mean they were at another table.

THERAPIST: And how would that feel? If they were laughing at someone else, I mean?

PATIENT: Well, it's not very nice but it wouldn't have bothered me so much.

THERAPIST: So, thinking over all the possibilities we listed, that they were sharing a joke, or remembering something funny, or planning something or even laughing at someone else. Thinking about all of those, how sure do you feel that they were absolutely positively laughing at you?

PATIENT: Not so sure I guess.

THERAPIST: Good. So imagine you're back in the lunchroom again tomorrow; and you see some guys laughing about something. Do you think you could go over all the options for what might be funny? How would you feel if you did that?

PATIENT: I probably wouldn't have to leave if I did that.

This example highlights the way anxious thoughts can trigger emotions and lead to avoidant behavior that prevent any actual testing of the veracity of the thoughts themselves. Children have an automatic interpretation of an ambiguous situation, fueled by the preexisting fear of ridicule and shame, which in turn leads to feelings of embarrassment and to their avoiding the potential for more such situations in the future (by not eating lunch in the public space anymore). With each day of continued avoidance the memory of the aversive experience is likely to become more distressing so that the possibility of returning to the lunchroom becomes more remote. What may have begun as a temporary solution becomes increasingly likely to be the permanent rule. By applying cognitive restructuring, the therapist is helping the patient to observe the way in which one particular thought has "hijacked" the cognitive process leading to particular results, while other thoughts could have different outcomes. Figure 4.1 illustrates some additional examples of cognitive restructuring.

A good way to involve a young child more actively in cognitive restructuring is to simulate a "boxing match" between the anxiety on the one hand and realistic thoughts on the other. Child and therapist, or child and parent, can battle it out and take turns representing either side in the match. By doing so, the negative automatic cognitions that many children will otherwise leave vague or ambiguous become explicated and the opportunity arises to challenge them with information on perspectives that the child would not otherwise access.

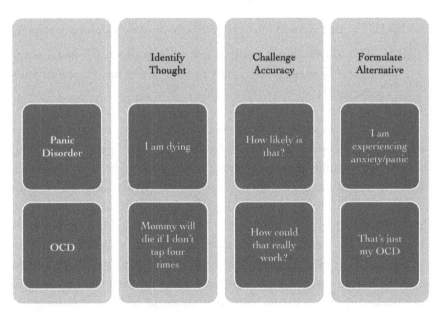

Figure 4.1 Two examples illustrating the process of cognitive restructuring for panic disorder and OCD

A typical "boxing match" might go something like this:

ANXIETY: You're going to be kidnapped from bed tonight. You definitely are [Pow! Anxiety landed a good one!]

REALITY: Kidnappings are really rare. They almost never happen like that at all. [Nice parry!]

ANXIETY: They'll come in the window and take you. You'll never see your parents again! [Anxiety throws another punch!]

REALITY: My parents lock the windows and doors at night; no one is likely to be able to come in. [Ooh. Nice defense! Keeping on your toes.]

ANXIETY: But they'll forget. You remember that story about the boy who was kidnapped. That could be you! [Anxiety is still fighting back.]

REALITY: That was just a story. In real life that is very unlikely. I never heard of anyone I know getting kidnapped. [Good! Just keep throwing punches like that!]

ANXIETY: But it could happen. [Anxiety definitely getting weaker!]

REALITY: Maybe, but it really is not realistic at all. It's just a scary thought. My parents know how to take care of me. [Beautiful! It's a knockout!]

Although the experience of stating such thoughts so explicitly may make some therapists uncomfortable or fear that they are "feeding the anxiety" rather than alleviating it, it is actually the avoidance of the thoughts that grants them most power. By allowing the child to play the role of anxiety or by basing the statements anxiety makes on things the child has said, the therapist can feel certain that even the most anxious thoughts are only ones that exist in the child's imagination anyway. In fact, most children feel immense relief at being allowed to voice their most scary thoughts and at finding an adult who not only is not shocked by them but is also quite unafraid of them. Limiting the conversation to only mild thoughts or less frightening ideas reinforces the feeling that the most disturbing thoughts actually do pose some risk to the child, rather than relegating them to their true role—that of things that have no power at all beyond making one somewhat uncomfortable for a while. The repeated stating of the anxiety-provoking thoughts in exercises such as these also serves as a kind of exposure to the thoughts themselves and has the effect that any exposure has—to desensitize the child to them and lessen the emotional reaction they provoke. This is soon felt in the child's decreased sensitivity to the content as the exercise is repeated. In Chapter 5 on behavioral interventions, we discuss exposure and desensitization and describe how this principle can be applied in creating "imagined exposures," in which the thoughts themselves serve as the stimulus to which the child becomes habituated.

Parents can practice cognitive restructuring at home with their child, creating not only more opportunities for progress but also sending the child some very important messages. First, the technique can create an alliance between parent and child that leaves anxiety in the role of a common enemy to overcome together. This is different from the potential situation of parents feeling like they and the child are on opposite sides of a battle. Parents' futile attempts to alleviate a child's anxiety through reassurance and protection can lead them to feel frustrated when those attempts don't work and can leave the child feeling misunderstood. By engaging together in cognitive restructuring, or other techniques described below, and by externalizing the problem through discussing "what anxiety says" rather than what "you're afraid of," parent and child stand united to overcome a common challenge.

It is important to stress that the child need not identify with the more realistic thoughts or believe them to be true for the positive effects of cognitive restructuring to take place. It is often useful to directly tell the children not to attempt to change their actual position, at least at first, but rather to concentrate on producing and stating the alternative cognitions in an almost artificial or pretend way. The benefits of restructuring are first felt in creating space for more than one potential scenario and in engaging children in directly addressing and challenging the anxiety rather than in actually shifting their position. Children who repeatedly say "But I don't really believe that," feeling that the "trick isn't working," can be praised for completing their role particularly well in having focused on producing the thoughts. In this way a sense of failure can be reframed as a success and motivation preserved.

Recruiting the Imagination (Guided Imagery)

As therapists we have often been quite astounded at the power that the imagination can have to alleviate even acute anxiety. The techniques described here, and many other similar ones, are so absurdly simple that time and again we are amazed at how powerful they can be. Perhaps the best way to understand the power of imagination in combating anxiety is to remember that ultimately it is always the imagination that is triggering the anxiety in the first place. After all, almost by definition when we are anxious we are imagining some negative outcome and feeling fear as a response. Anxiety is based entirely on our ability to imagine negative events and thereby to dread them. It is not surprising that so many parents of children suffering from anxiety describe their children as having particularly rich imaginations as well.

For many children with anxiety disorders the real problem seems to be actually not recognizing the role imagination plays in their fears. Instead of identifying the thought as a figment of imagination, the child attempts to "fix" the problem as if it were a real-world issue. This is particularly true of children suffering from obsessive-compulsive disorder. In OCD children may experience repeated catastrophic thoughts and perform rituals so as to ensure that the thoughts do not materialize. In essence, they are trying to impose a real-world solution on an imagination-world problem. Not surprisingly, this does not work well while treating the problem in its own true domain, of cognitions and ideations, might.

One good way to explain this idea to children and parents is to contrast real-life problems with imagination problems:

> Imagine you are being attacked by a bandit. He's aiming a gun at you and threatening to kill you! Trying to "imagine" your way out of that situation is not a good idea. You have a real problem and you need to do something real about, like running away. But now think about your imaginary fears. Say for example that you are afraid of a ghost. You can run as fast as you like but the ghost will keep up with you because he's in your head! In this case trying to fix the problem in "the real world" can't work because the ghost lives inside your head. So you need an "inside" solution, something that can change your imagination. The fears that occur in an anxiety disorder are imagined fears and the imagination is a powerful tool for changing them — better than trying to run away in the real world.

Watching your thoughts leave—there are many ways to perform this exercise and here are two of our favorites:

The train station in the mind: Imagine that your mind is like a train station. Your thoughts are going to be the trains that pass through the station. Imagine yourself in the station. You might want to look around and notice some of the features of the station, like its color or the location of the ticket vendors or perhaps an information desk. You are standing in the station and all is quiet. A few people are scattered here and there and the faint smell of engine fumes is in the air but the atmosphere is generally quiet and relaxed. Then a train approaches the station. It brings with it great plumes of dark black smoke that billow out of its chimney. It makes a great metallic screeching noise that grates unpleasantly on the ears and crowds of loud bustling people spill out, shattering the calm environment that existed before. You would like to prevent this from happening but you cannot. After all, standing on train tracks and trying to block an incoming train is only going to get you crushed. There is no way you can block it. But if you only wait a very few minutes you will find you don't really need to. Soon the people leave the station to go on their way. The train pulls out of the station and you watch it drive away, taking all the smoke and smell and noise with it. As it goes farther and farther away the station returns to the relaxed way it was before. You didn't need to do anything at all. Just by waiting, it all went away.[1]

Floating balloons: Imagine a field—a green, wide field stretched as far as you can see. And over the field the sky is blue and clear like on a really nice day. Now imagine a hot air balloon floating over this field gently drifting from over you and across the field, heading off toward the horizon. In the basket hanging from under the balloon I want you to place a thought that's been bothering you or that is troubling you right now. It could be any thought—any—you can put it there any way you like. You could imagine writing it on paper and placing that there, or imagine a picture of your thought in the basket or just imagine that you

---

[1]A variation on this exercise call for the children to imagine that their negative thought is on the train in some way, for example, as a picture on the side of the train, and to watch the thought being brought into the station with the train and then growing farther and farther away as it leaves.

have placed your thought there in some way. Now watch as the balloon drifts gently away from you, going farther and farther and taking your thought with it. Soon you can hardly see the balloon or the thought at all and then it disappears entirely. Now if you like you can summon another balloon and put another thought on it. Watch as it, too, drifts slowly away over the field. You can put as many thoughts as you like or you can put the same thought again if it still is bothering you and watch until it disappears again.

PARENT GUIDANCE

Parents, too, have negative and catastrophic cognitions relating to their child's anxiety disorder, and addressing these unrealistic thoughts will be an important aspect of the cognitive work. Among the thoughts that race through the minds of parents observing their child experiencing an attack of anxiety are cognitions such as:

- He's so sensitive, he probably won't hold up!
- If I don't help him right now, something terrible will happen to him!
- I have to save him!
- You can't let such a small child suffer so much!

Just as children are tasked with identifying their maladaptive beliefs and substituting them for more realistic ones, parents, too, can engage in cognitive restructuring. Here are some more factually accurate and more confidence-inspiring thoughts that parents have used to reduce their own level of panic:

- She's sensitive, but she has tolerance, too.
- If I run to save him, I'm hurting him, not helping!
- She is not in danger!
- If I rush to protect him I'm adding my own fear on top of his!
- This will subside soon, and she'll still be okay.
- I want to be able to praise him getting through it!
- By controlling my own reaction—I give him the chance to control his.

Just like the child, the parent does not have to completely identify with the alternative cognitions to practice cognitive restructuring. Stating the thoughts clearly and explicitly will usually have the effect of reducing anxiety and alleviating the parental sense of urgency even when the parent remains unconvinced that the thoughts are factually correct.

By engaging in cognitive restructuring themselves, the parents not only allow children time to self-regulate their own inner state without reliance on external soothing or reassurance, they also model adaptive behavior for their child. For this reason we encourage parents not to hide their experience from their child but rather to be quite open about it. If a child asks: *Didn't it bother you to see me so upset?* The parent does not need to feel compelled to hide the turmoil of their own experience but rather can view it as an opportunity to express support by combining acceptance of anxiety with the need for coping: *Of course, it did! It was terrible to see how anxious you were feeling! But I was counting on you to get through it, and you know what? You did! I'm so proud of both of us!*

The parents' focus on their own anxious thoughts or scenarios can aid in another kind of frustration they might feel in their relationship with their anxious child as well. Many parents discover that when they attempt to redirect the children's thought patterns in more positive or confident directions, the children seem to "dig in" to their negative views more obstinately than ever. The parents may be surprised to discover that their suggestions have brought about the opposite of what they intended and that the children are resisting their suggestions or becoming immune to them. This experience is particularly powerful among parents of adolescents, although it is not uncommon with younger children as well. By shifting focus away from the attempt to correct children's thoughts and instead focusing on their own, parents can learn to relate differently to the anxiety. For example, a mother might say to her child: "I realized I was wrong when I thought you were so sensitive, that you couldn't handle the anxiety!" or "I've learned that I can restrain myself when you are stressed" or "I've discovered that my tension, and maybe also yours, does not constantly rise, it rises at first and then goes back down!" In these examples parents have abandoned the preaching tone that many children find unhelpful and are illustrating their own struggle instead. There is no need to repeat these remarks often, creating a feeling of oblique sermonizing or nagging. Through self-restraint the parent is sending the message that "I practice what I preach" and "I can only come to conclusions for myself, not for you!"

Parents should also be aware of the issue of cognitive avoidance and take care not to implicitly or explicitly convey to the child that thinking the thoughts, or mentioning them, is wrong and should be avoided. Children who sense that their fears cause their parents discomfort to the extent that they are expected not to mention them, or not to even think them, cannot help but experience even more fear—and consequently even more thoughts. Often parents will unwittingly play into children's natural sense that their thoughts have a magical power to do harm in the world. For example, a child may say to her mother "Last night I dreamt of you dying and my being all alone" and a parent may naturally respond: "Hush, don't even speak of such a thing" or simply "Put that out of your mind." These responses can inadvertently instill a fear of thinking the thing for fear of causing it to happen and trap a child in a loop of frustrating failed attempts to control anxious thoughts. A less natural but probably more helpful response might be: "I'm sure that made you very uncomfortable, but it really doesn't mean anything at all" or "No one can control their dreams so it doesn't even pay to try." In this way, not only are parents sending a message that does not encourage futile attempts at avoidance but they are also telling the children that they have no guilt in thinking (or dreaming) about a thing because they are not in control of their own thoughts.

The message that a child is not in control of his or her own thoughts is one that parents should emphasize often. For many children, especially those who tend to be overly or rigidly scrupulous, the act of thinking a thing can mean that they have done something wrong or will in the future.

A 12-year-old boy was watching a movie about a serial killer when he had the disconcerting thought, "What if I were to become a serial killer in the future." He immediately was filled with remorse at having thought such a thing but remained troubled that the thought indicated that there lurked inside of him a dark wish to kill others. From that moment he repeatedly had thoughts about becoming a killer and gradually became almost convinced that this was likely to happen in the future. His parents noticed that he was now unwilling to remain alone in the room with his younger sister, and after querying him about it for some time he admitted that he was acting for her own protection as he was sure he could kill her if the two were left alone.

Parents faced with such a scenario can easily be understood if they do not wish to leave their children alone together, but responding in this way is almost certain to elevate the anxiety even more. A healthier approach would be one that emphasizes the quirkiness of the human brain and the individual's inability to control unwanted thoughts. An important point to emphasize to parents is that intrusive thoughts do not indicate "secret wishes," they indicate *fears*. Children have recurrent thoughts about the things they fear the most (see tunnel vision earlier), and interpreting these as a warning sign can only cause more fear to become attached to the thought.

Another lesson for parents that stems from understanding the impact of anxiety on cognition is the futility of trying to "talk a child out of her fears," especially when the child is acutely anxious. Many parents will have had the experience of seeing their child panicking about a realistically innocuous situation and trying to make them "see sense." This kind of attempt is usually futile at best and harmful at worst. The tunnel vision effect of anxiety on the child's thought processes makes it difficult to attend to the parents' words and the elevated risk assessment can make it hard to think rationally about the larger scheme of things or to take into account realistic information. Unfortunately, many parents will respond to this difficulty by trying to make the message more forceful, as if to break through the children's wall of anxiety that seems to be blocking them from seeing the truth of what the parent is saying. This can easily lead to a strained communication and to frustration for all involved.

By helping parents to appreciate the effect that anxiety has on cognitive functioning, such stressful experiences can be reduced. Parents who understand that their child is not "stubbornly refusing to listen" and does not "want to remain anxious" will be better prepared to maintain their own calm. Additionally, the importance of discussing the problem when the child is calm becomes more apparent. Often a parent will talk about a child's anxiety almost exclusively when the child is most anxious. This is natural as this is when the problem seems most pressing and hardest to ignore. Or perhaps the parents fear triggering anxiety by raising the topic when the child is actually feeling better. However, this also dictates that the discussion must always be held under the negative influence of acute anxiety and can lead parents to see their child as less collaborative and more obstinate than is actually the case.

In summary, parent guidance can augment the cognitive work done with a child by highlighting the cognitive impact of anxiety, teaching and implementing cognitive skills and strategies, and helping parents to model more adaptive coping for the child.

REFERENCES

Amir, N., Elias, J., Klumpp, H., & Przeworski, A. (2003). Attentional bias to threat in social phobia: Facilitated processing of threat or difficulty disengaging attention from threat? *Behaviour Research and Therapy*, *41*(11), 1325–1335. doi:10.1016/s0005–7967 (03)00039–1

Angie, A. D., Connelly, S., Waples, E. P., & Kligyte, V. (2011). The influence of discrete emotions on judgement and decision-making: A meta-analytic review. *Cognition and Emotion*, *25*(8), 1393–1422.

Bar-Haim, Y., Lamy, D., & Glickman, S. (2005). Attentional bias in anxiety: A behavioral and ERP study. *Brain and Cognition*, *59*(1), 11–22. doi:10.1016/j.bandc.2005.03.005

Beck, A. T. (2008). The evolution of the cognitive model of depression and its neurobiological correlates. [Peer Reviewed]. *American Journal of Psychiatry*, *165*(8), 969–977. doi:10.1176/appi.ajp.2008.08050721

Beck, A. T., Emery, G., & Greenberg, R. L. (2005). *Anxiety disorders and phobias: A cognitive perspective* (15th anniversary ed.). Cambridge, MA: Basic Books.

Fox, E., Russo, R., Bowles, R., & Dutton, K. (2001). Do threatening stimuli draw or hold visual attention in subclinical anxiety? *Journal of Experimental Psychology: General*, *130*(4), 681–700. doi:10.1037/0096–3445.130.4.681

References

Libby, S., Reynolds, S., Derisley, J., & Clark, S. (2004). Cognitive appraisals in young people with obsessive-compulsive disorder. *Journal of Child Psychology and Psychiatry, 45*(6), 1076–1084. doi:http://dx.doi.org/10.1111/j.1469-7610.2004.t01-1-00300.x

Lira Yoon, K., & Zinbarg, R. E. (2007). Threat is in the eye of the beholder: Social anxiety and the interpretation of ambiguous facial expressions. *Behaviour Research and Therapy, 45*(4), 839–847. doi:10.1016/j.brat.2006.05.004

Loewenstein, G. F., Hsee, C. K., Weber, E. U., & Welch, N. (2001). Risk as feelings. *Psychological Bulletin, 127*(2), 267–286.

Logan, A. C., & Goetsch, V. L. (1993). Attention to external threat cues in anxiety states. *Clinical Psychology Review, 13*(6), 541–559. doi:10.1016/0272-7358(93)90045-n

MacLeod, C., & Cohen, I. L. (1993). Anxiety and the interpretation of ambiguity: A text comprehension study. *Journal of Abnormal Psychology, 102*(2), 238–247. doi:10.1037/0021-843x.102.2.238

Maner, J. K., & Schmidt, N. B. (2006). The role of risk avoidance in anxiety. *Behavior Therapy, 37*(2), 181–189. doi:10.1016/j.beth.2005.11.003

Monk, C. S., Nelson, E. E., McClure, E. B., Mogg, K., Bradley, B. P., Leibenluft, E., . . . Pine, D. S. (2006). Ventrolateral prefrontal cortex activation and attentional bias in response to angry faces in adolescents with generalized anxiety disorder. *American Journal of Psychiatry, 163*(6), 1091–1097.

Moradi, A. R., Taghavi, R., Neshat-Doost, H. T., Yule, W., & Dalgleish, T. (2000). Memory bias for emotional information in children and adolescents with posttraumatic stress disorder: A preliminary study. *Journal of Anxiety Disorders, 14*(5), 521–534. doi:10.1016/s0887-6185(00)00037-2

Rees, C. S., Draper, M., & Davis, M. C. (2010). The relationship between magical thinking, thought-action fusion and obsessive-compulsive symptoms. *International Journal of Cognitive Therapy, 3*(3), 304–311. http://dx.doi.org/10.1521/ijct.2010.3.3.304

Roy, A. K., Vasa, R. A., Bruck, M., Mogg, K., Bradley, B. P., Sweeney, M., . . . Team, C. (2008). Attention bias toward threat in pediatric anxiety disorders. *Journal of the American Academy of Child & Adolescent Psychiatry, 47*(10), 1189–1196.

Russo, R., Whittuck, D., Roberson, D., Dutton, K., Georgiou, G., & Fox, E. (2006). Mood-congruent free recall bias in anxious individuals is not a consequence of response bias. *Memory, 14*(4), 393–399.

Teachman, B. A. (2005). Information processing and anxiety sensitivity: Cognitive vulnerability to panic reflected in interpretation and memory biases. *Cognitive Therapy and Research, 29*(4), 479–499. doi:10.1007/s10608–005–0627–5

CHAPTER FIVE

Behavioral Tools for Treating Anxiety

The most "active ingredient" in treating childhood anxiety is exposure. By gradually and repeatedly facing previously avoided anxiety-provoking situations in a supportive environment a child becomes desensitized to the stimulus and anxiety is immensely and reliably reduced. The trick is getting the child to participate in the exposures.

Key points in this chapter:

- Anxiety can lead to significant changes in a child's behavior—primarily causing avoidance and increasing the need for control.
- Exposure and desensitization is a powerful tool in reducing anxiety and decreasing avoidance.
- Exposures should usually be gradual, prolonged, and repeated.
- Helpful tools for parents to support their child's behavioral changes.
- A plan for getting children to sleep in their own bed.

THE BEHAVIORAL ELEMENT OF ANXIETY

Experiencing anxiety effects behavior in a number of important ways, and understanding them is a key component in creating effective strategies for modifying the behavior and channeling it in more adaptive directions. We begin by describing two of the major behavioral ramifications of anxiety in children and then turn to designing and implementing successful behavioral interventions.

Avoidance

The foremost behavioral outcome of anxiety is avoidance. Avoidance refers to any steps a child may take to minimize contact with an anxiety-provoking stimulus. As in other aspects of anxiety, it is useful to remember "what anxiety is for" when thinking about avoidance. In fulfilling its primary role of protecting the organism from danger, anxiety works to prevent the child from encountering potentially hazardous situations. Anxiety would be an ineffective system indeed if it caused people to take more risks rather than less. Some people take pleasure in stimulating their anxiety response by experiencing thrilling or frightening situations—but this is usually only pleasurable when the overall appraisal is that the situation is safe and the anxiety is tightly framed in an otherwise nonthreatening situation (few people would enjoy a roller coaster ride if they did not have confidence that it was reasonably safe).

One useful way to explain to children and parents the utility of avoidance in anxiety is by comparing it to pain:

> Everyone hates feeling pain—of course they do, it hurts! So why do we feel pain at all? It helps to know when something is wrong so that we can fix it. For example, imagine you were leaning against a really hot pot and your hand was going to get burned. You would feel pretty strong pain and you would move your hand really quickly! The pain would have been unpleasant but because of that you would have acted swiftly to eliminate it. If it felt really good, or even just neutral, you might have left your hand there longer and perhaps have been seriously injured. Anxiety is very similar except instead of hurting because of something that is already causing injury, it tells us to be careful of something that **might** hurt us. It's like pain for injury that has not happened yet and it wants to help make sure that it won't. That's why if you know a pot is hot your anxiety will make sure you don't touch it in the first place. If it felt really good we might want to do lots of things that would hurt us instead of avoiding them.

Avoidance Reinforces Anxiety

When a child suffers from an anxiety disorder the natural tendency to avoid the stimuli that trigger the anxiety can have very serious repercussions. One of the results of continually avoiding a harmless situation is that the individual never has the opportunity to learn that the anxiety is actually misplaced. For example, a child who believes that ladybugs bite with a terrible painful bite may run hysterically at the sight of a ladybug—and will never learn that they are actually quite amicable. Children who are convinced that they will get trapped forever if they enter an elevator will always walk the stairs and never experience a safe elevator journey.

A related phenomenon occurs when children escape from frightening— but not actually dangerous—situations. They may experience a strong sense of relief when the avoidance is complete. The substitution of fear with relief is a powerful negative reinforcement that promotes the repetition of the same behavior in the future. Often, children will take their successful "escape" as proof that the anxiety was actually well founded. In the case of the elevator, for example, children will attribute their repeatedly getting safely to their destination as proof that taking the stairs was the correct strategy—ignoring the possibility that they would have done equally well riding. Recognizing the powerful drive to escape from the unpleasant internal arousal triggered by anxiety has led some therapeutic approaches to focus on increasing the patient's ability to withstand distress rather than on directly minimizing the distress caused by given stimuli or situations (Hofmann, Sawyer, Witt, & Oh, 2010; Waltz & Hayes, 2010).

Safety Behaviors—Active Avoidance

Although some instances of avoidance are obvious and direct (i.e., "I won't go to the sleepover because I'm afraid"), other times avoidance can take a more subtle and less easily recognized form. An example of this is the frequent use of safety behaviors to aid children in managing a situation they deem to be alarming. A child suffering from agoraphobia may not avoid places altogether but may insist on being accompanied to different locations so as to avoid the chance of experiencing a panic attack while alone. Even more subtly children may take water bottles with them everywhere they go, perform ritualized behaviors in a variety of contexts, or only preface everything they say with "I think" so as to avoid making a mistake.

Avoidance is usually thought of in the negative, as the absence of action. Parents may list all the things their child *won't* do when asked to describe avoidant behaviors, but safety behaviors include a host of actions a child may actively engage in, so as to avoid feeling anxious. Children with separation anxiety may call their parents multiple times a day on the phone to as to escape the feeling of anxiety triggered by their absence, and children with a fear of dogs may choose to walk on only one side of a street because they believe the other one is dangerous. Some children spend considerable amounts of time searching for bugs in their room before going to sleep because they wish to avoid the anxiety of worrying about an insect crawling on them at night.

Engaging in such safety behaviors has the potential to maintain anxiety and to undermine the desensitization that would otherwise be achieved by exposure to the anxiety provoking situations. For example, in a study of individuals with panic disorder with agoraphobia, the participants were asked to engage in an activity that they found very difficult, such as walking outside or entering a department store. Subjects who were instructed to refrain from safety-seeking behaviors showed significantly greater reductions in anxiety following the exposure than those who were not instructed to do so (Salkovskis, Clark, Hackmann, Wells, & Gelder, 1999). Similarly, among patients with social phobia, reducing safety behaviors during exposures to social situations increases their efficacy whereas engaging in them appears to maintain the anxiety (Eun-Jung, 2005; Wells et al., 1995).

Understanding, mapping, and addressing safety behaviors can be an important part of overcoming an anxiety disorder and often requires specifically targeted questions. Safety behaviors can sometimes be hard to differentiate from stages in gradual exposure (Thwaites & Freeston, 2005) and at times may be important in allowing a child to participate in a situation that would otherwise be avoided entirely. However, they should be seen as a temporary stage at most, in overcoming the disorder, rather than a lasting solution. The main reason for this is that by continuing to engage in excessive safety behaviors, children continually reinforce their own belief in the danger of the stimulus. By telling themselves "I can do this—because of the safety behavior," children will not gain the sense that "I can do this—because I no longer feel afraid." Just as exposures should be undertaken gradually (as we describe later in this chapter), the relinquishment of safety behaviors also need to be undertaken gradually so that complete avoidance does not replace partial avoidance, but the therapist should not confuse exposure with "safety mediated exposure."

Generalization

A phenomenon well known to researchers of behavior and learning (in both animals and humans) is that of generalization. In the basic paradigm a response that comes to be associated with a certain stimulus will often be generalized to other similar or related stimuli. This is particularly true of the fear response, although the networks of association can be hard to trace for any give individual or disorder (Dymond & Roche, 2009; Lissek et al., 2005). Once again, keeping in mind the basic nature of anxiety as a danger-avoidance system makes the principle easily understandable. The person who narrowly escapes death by bear mauling is unlikely to come away from the experience with the idea that *that particular bear* is dangerous. Rather he will (hopefully) learn that *bears are dangerous* or perhaps even generalize the conclusion to all large wild animals. A similar phenomenon occurs with much less helpful effects in anxiety disorders:

> When I first met Edmund he was 7 years old and suffering from a severe phobia of dogs. His fear was so intense that he had developed a set of avoidance-precautions that he took to escape ever triggering it. Not only would he not agree to be in the vicinity of a dog, he refused to see pictures of dogs in books, watch any movies that featured dogs, or hear a story about dogs. The very mention of the word *dog* caused him to go red in the face, wave his arms dramatically, and object loudly until the topic was dropped and the perpetrator promised not to repeat the offense.
>
> His mother described the process by which this situation had been shaped: "At first he wouldn't go to the park because of all the dogs there, then he said he wanted us to drive him everywhere because walking on the sidewalk he constantly imagined a dog jumping on him. After that he began to avoid certain films like *101 Dalmatians* that had dogs in them.

He started asking when I went to the library if I was going to get 'a dog book' and things have just gotten worse and worse. I'm afraid soon he won't be able to leave home at all."

Rapid Fear Learning

Most learning takes time, often a lot of time. Repetition, rehearsal, and review all go into helping to consolidate the neural connections that constitute learning. But fear learning can happen quickly—sometimes with just a single instance sufficing to teach avoidance that can last a lifetime (Rescorla, 1988). This may be particularly true of certain kinds of fears. Children who are exposed to traumatic situations can develop posttraumatic stress disorder characterized by long-term avoidance, in addition to intrusive ideation about the distressing trigger. Children who undergo less dramatic experiences can also develop fear and avoidance after a single trial, given the right situation. Many people will have the experience of eating an unfamiliar food and subsequently becoming ill or feeling sick. This generally occurs through simple coincidence as both of those eventualities are quite common in the life of most children. But the temporal pairing of Event A (eating a certain food) and Event B (becoming sick) can create an association that will lead to prolonged, and at times extreme, avoidance. The prevalence of such taste aversions in the general population has been found to be very high (Logue, 1985; Logue, Ophir, & Strauss, 1981).

> Dahlia was 11 years old when she became sick with a stomach virus. She experienced strong nausea and threw up violently a number of times. Earlier that day she had eaten a corndog for the first time. When a relative mentioned the corndog the next day in passing, she became acutely nauseous and ran to throw up again. Soon after that the very mention of corn itself was enough to trigger sensations of nausea and severe anxiety and she became careful not to come into contact with anything made of corn. When she first came for treatment she would not allow her parents to buy anything that had corn listed in the ingredients, including items containing corn flour, corn starch, corn syrup, and dextrose corn sugar! "Do you know how hard it is to shop for a family without buying anything containing corn?" her mother asked.

Dahlia was demonstrating both of the phenomena described above. Rapid fear learning accounted for her intense avoidance after a single episode of becoming sick following the experience of eating a corndog, and the powerful natural tendency to generalization in anxiety had led her to broaden the boundaries of her avoidance until it encompassed anything remotely related to corn.

Control

Another important behavioral shift typical of children experiencing heightened levels of anxiety is an increase in the need for control (Moulding & Kyrios, 2006; Pervin, 1963). Control can be thought of in many different ways, but for our purposes we can define control as an individual child's ability to predict and to influence events. Children who do not have the ability to influence what is about to happen, for example, children being taken to a doctor's office whether they want to or not, may still have the ability to predict how the visit will go. That child will still have a greater sense of control than one who not only cannot decide what is going to happen but also has no way of predicting it. Any information that further adds to those capacities, to know and to influence what is in store, increases control, and any circumstances that diminish them reduce the overall control the child will experience.

> Consider a child who is afraid of burglars and whose parents are thinking of going out for the evening and getting a babysitter. Total control for that child might be the ability to say to his parents "No, I don't want you to go because it makes me nervous" and for them to say home. Barring that, the child is likely to ask numerous questions aimed at increasing his overall sense of control: "Where will you be going?"; "When will you get back?" and so on. The more information supplied, the greater the overall sense of perceived control.

Anxiety heightens a child's need for control by emphasizing the potential for negative events and outcomes (Weems, Silverman, Rapee, & Pina, 2003). Children with little tendency toward anxiety may feel that most situations are likely to be positive or within their ability to cope, and as a result it is less important to know exactly *how* a situation will end well. By contrast, anxious children who view many situations as potentially dangerous and their own capacity to forbear as far from guaranteed, may feel compelled to ensure that things go exactly according to plan. Any deviation from plans and expectations can trigger fearful thoughts and feelings and the need for control is a natural consequence of this worldview.

In our experience, many parents describe their anxious child as being "controlling," "bossy," or even "a tyrant" for these reasons. However, confusing a child's need for control with an inherent and negative personality trait is likely to be both inaccurate and unhelpful. In a large international survey that addressed the most controlling behaviors of children with obsessive-compulsive disorder, 88% of experts in the field agreed that the behaviors were more likely to be secondary to the child's anxiety (and to disappear when the anxiety disorder improved) rather than to reflect an innate trait toward controlling or disruptive behavior (Lebowitz, Vitulano, Mataix-Cols, & Leckman, 2011). Helping parents to frame the child's behavior in the context of anxiety-driven need for control can help to reframe the parents' role as well. Rather than a need to "resist the child's demands" or to "show her who's in charge," parents can see themselves as working to increase a child's ability to withstand uncertainty or to handle the lack of control that is inherent to living in the world. In the section of this book that deals with parent-based treatment (see Chapter 11) we discuss some innovative ways for dealing with the extreme control imposed by some anxious children on their families, but for most parents simply understanding why anxiety is making their child act in a controlling fashion can be the most important step. By helping parents to grasp this idea the therapist can release them from the false dilemma of "Do I give in or do I stand up to her?" In fact, the choice is not between submission and resistance but between reinforcing children's belief that they cannot cope with anything less than perfect control and promoting their ability to navigate the unpredictable waters of life.

BEHAVIORAL TOOLS FOR WORKING WITH THE CHILD

The most important element in the treatment of childhood anxiety disorders is the behavioral component—exposures to the previously avoided stimuli. The premise behind exposure is simple, reliable, and familiar for all children — repeated exposure leads to desensitization. All children will have a rudimentary understanding of this principle, attained through their own experience of life and can easily grasp its applicability to fears and anxiety. For some years I have made it my practice to ask children suffering from anxiety what advice they would give to a friend who was also suffering from some fear. For younger children I often tell a story about a friend of mine who cannot come visit me because I have a cat and he is terrified of cats; so scared, in fact, that he cannot even enter my home. For older children I suggest that they imagine that a friend of theirs was suffering from a fear that was interfering with their ability to live normally. I am often puzzled when I hear colleagues say that CBT cannot be applied to very young children because in the years that I have been asking their advice on treating anxiety, the majority have always suggested to me that the friend attempt behavioral exposures in one form or another. In other words, even very young children, starting from around age 5 at the latest, are not only capable of understanding the principles of exposures but of independently formulating them as a cure for unwarranted anxiety.

Exposures can be implemented in any number of ways, but some principles are common to most successful plans and together constitute useful guidelines for planning and executing effective exposures. A good plan ensures that exposures are gradual, repeated, and prolonged.

Gradual Exposure

One rule that almost never fails to hold true is that in planning exposures the longer way is actually the shorter way. Attempts to make quick progress or to take large steps forward will often backfire, resulting in a reluctance to do any further exposures. The risk of feelings of disappointment or of failure that can result from premature attempts to take on large challenges outweighs the potential for satisfaction in having accomplished rapid progress. In fact, the ideal situation for therapists to be in is that of the child pulling them forward and urging them to go more quickly, a much better situation than being the one pushing the child forward.

Exposure Hierarchy

To ensure a gradual process that is suited to the specific reactions of a given child, the therapist and the patient create together an *exposure hierarchy*. The hierarchy lists various steps that children will take in gradually overcoming their fear. The first steps on the hierarchy should be easy enough to ensure success. Therapists should be adamant about not starting with exposures that are too hard and should attempt to choose initial exposures that trigger a degree of fear well beneath what might be considered the child's maximum tolerance level. This is important to ensure that the child will be successful in withstanding the fear and to allow for progress to be made after the initial step. Children who take on a first exposure that challenges them to the utmost extent of their ability may feel that further steps afterward are impossible. Figures 5.1 and 5.2 illustrate exposure hierarchies.

It may be useful to have children rate the degree of fear they believe that each step on the projected hierarchy will trigger. This is helpful in ordering the steps from least hard to most difficult, but the actual ratings should be taken as no more than a guess and not assumed to represent

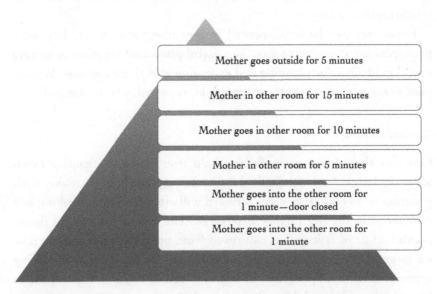

Mother goes outside for 5 minutes

Mother in other room for 15 minutes

Mother goes in other room for 10 minutes

Mother in other room for 5 minutes

Mother goes into the other room for 1 minute—door closed

Mother goes into the other room for 1 minute

Figure 5.1 Example of an exposure hierarchy for a child with separation anxiety.

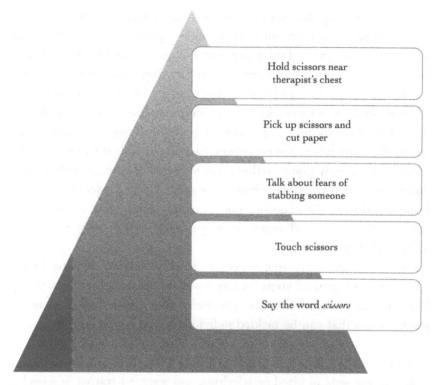

Figure 5.2 Example of an exposure hierarchy for a child with OCD and aggressive obsessions.

what the child will actually experience. When anxious, most children will rate any step as being considerably more difficult than it will actually prove to be. This is partly due to the extreme avoidance that has already become a part of the child's life. Through the continuous process of generalization many children will have come to avoid any number of situations as precautions against feeling anxious. For many of them, actually coming face-to-face with the stimulus will be almost anti-climactic in that it will only provoke moderate anxiety. Rather than trying to convince children that an exposure will be less difficult than they believe, these situations present opportunities to teach children that they can overcome even experiences they think of as very difficult. It is also an opportunity to learn another important lesson — that anxiety "cheats" them by making them think that actions will be much harder than they prove to be.

Often by taking into consideration various parameters that make the exposures easier or more difficult, a single exposure can be repeated in many varying degrees of difficulty. For example, a child with separation anxiety may choose a challenge such as "staying home alone while my parents go out for half an hour." This can easily be expanded into many different steps on a hierarchy by adjusting variables such as the time of day when the exposure is performed (nighttime may be harder than during the day); where the parents go (waiting outside the house may be easier than actually going farther away); degree of contact with parents during the exposure (are phone calls allowed?); presence of safety behaviors during the exposure (i.e., leaving all the lights on or having the television on), and many other parameters that vary with each individual child.

Often, the most creative aspect in treating anxiety will be in the formulation of gradual steps for exposure. With enough creativity, *any* fear and *any* avoided situation can be broken down into a series of smaller steps that can be tackled individually.

Jordan was 14 and had needle/blood phobia. He had been known to faint at even the sight of blood on television, and when his teacher in school had explained the workings of an MRI he had swooned immediately. Now Jordan had come to treatment because he wanted to participate in a school activity that his doctor was unwilling to sanction unless he had a full physical examination including some blood work. Caught between his fear and his desire to participate he decided, with his parents, to give behavioral therapy a try. Jordan listened attentively to my explanations about anxiety, behavioral therapy, exposures, and desensitization and then said, "But how can we take blood gradually? Either you prick me with a needle or you don't right?" We decided to skip normal protocol and jump right into creating a gradual sequence of exposures in our first session. We discussed many situations that could elicit anxiety on a widely ranging scale of severity. Seeing a hypodermic needle would be mildly distressing but holding one would be more so; watching a video of someone giving blood would be tremendously anxiety provoking he estimated, but watching a cartoon of the same would only cause mild discomfort. Jordan came to see that there were many steps we could take before he actually had to undergo his blood test. Over the next weeks we worked on many of these, and when the time came for him to do "the big one," to actually have blood taken from him, we broke that down into gradual steps as well. First, he underwent all the preparation such as rolling up his shirtsleeve, having his arm sanitized, and a rubber tourniquet tied around it. Next time he repeated those steps but this time a needle was actually touched to his arm. Only after he was comfortable with all these situations and no longer responded with anxiety or fainting did he actually have blood drawn.

Repeated Exposure

Repetition is a key ingredient in successfully treating anxiety. It is repetition, which will turn an exposure from something children have been able to survive into the kind of nonevent that will signal their desensitization. A common mistake is to proceed too rapidly from one successfully accomplished exposure to the next step on the hierarchy. In fact, a specific exposure should almost never be performed only once. After having successfully completed a certain step, children have gained confidence in their ability to withstand that level of anxiety. But they usually will not yet have learned that the step does not need to evoke the anxious sensations at all. By repeating the behavior numerous times, the sensation of anxiety will be replaced by one that approximates boredom, and children will have learned that they hold the key to transforming an exposure into a nonanxiety provoking situation. In this context, too, it is much better to have the child urging the process forward, eager to take on bigger challenges or move on to the next thing, than for the therapist to be the one spurring the child on before he or she feels prepared.

Prolonged Exposure

The third element of most successful exposures is duration. By allowing time for the anxiety to subside before any action is taken to escape from the situation, children can come to find themselves in the usually stressful situation—but absent the stress. This is not likely to happen unless there is sufficient time for the anxiety to peak, taper off, and recede. For most exposures this process will take between 15 and 25 minutes, with the maximum anxiety occurring early in the process. However, some children will not undertake an exposure for such a lengthy period of time and it is far more productive to allow children to

87

set the length of time they are willing to undergo than to attempt to force longer exposures on a reluctant child. Such an attempt is really only likely to replace their initial, albeit partial, willingness with a stubborn resistance, which will probably extend even to the originally agreeable assignment.

When a child is unwilling to embark on a prolonged exposure, the best alternative is usually to attempt shorter ones instead. Although these short exposures (sometimes less than a minute long) may not be as effective in desensitizing to the stimuli as longer ones would be, they will provide the first steps on the ladder and encourage the child to go on. Often a child will be surprised at the relatively low level of anxiety experienced during the brief exposure and thereafter may be much more willing to lengthen the process. The main thing the therapist should keep in mind is that by doing *any* exposure, even a seemingly ineffective one, the child is taking a major step forward. By agreeing to participate in the exposure, children are allying themselves with the therapist against the anxiety and taking the first step to standing up to anxiety. That first step is usually the most difficult one to take and the next may follow naturally in its wake.

Some situations naturally seem to take less time to complete, and the therapist will need to employ creativity in prolonging the exposure to attain desensitization. The case of the child who fears riding in an elevator is a classic example. The average elevator ride usually lasts no longer than 30 seconds, with the entire duration of the stay in the elevator taking less than a minute. For the purpose of exposure, however, it will be important to stay inside much longer. We have traveled up and down buildings repeatedly going from lobby to penthouse and back again over and over so as to reach the point where a child is no longer anxious.

Cognitive Exposure

Another way to target anxious thoughts, different from cognitive restructuring described in Chapter 4, is through cognitive exposure. In this case, rather than challenging the accuracy of the thoughts or formulating alternatives, thinking about the anxiety-provoking scenario becomes a kind of exposure and the ability of the thought to evoke a powerful emotional response is gradually diminished. This can be explained to children in the following way:

Think of the scariest movie you ever saw, or even one you would never see, but that you know about, something like *Nightmare on Elm Street*. Now maybe you would never watch that movie because it is so frightening. But imagine that one night, for some unfathomable reason, you were all alone at home and you decided to watch it. You would probably be terrified the whole way through, and you might want to cover your eyes or turn it off and race to hide under the covers. But just imagine that you didn't turn it off and somehow you watched the whole thing all the way to the end. When the movie was finished you'd probably be completely jumpy and afraid and you might want to turn on all the lights and double-lock all the doors. But what if instead of that you rewound the movie all the way to the beginning and started watching it again. This time the movie would probably still seem really scary, but it might be just a little bit less terrifying because at least you know what's coming. So you watch the whole thing through to the end again. And when it's over? You start it again! And you watch it all the way through. And then you do it again. And again! Say you did that 10 times. How would you be feeling during the 10th time? Would you be terrified? Would you still jump when something startling happens? More likely you would be feeling pretty bored! After all, how many times can the same movie scare you? In fact, you might even fall asleep! Imagine, falling asleep while *Nightmare on Elm Street* is playing right in front of you! When you started that would have seemed like an impossibility, something that could never happen. But by watching it over and over, and not turning it off or running away, you would have changed it from scary to boring. The same exact thing can happen with thoughts. When you have a frightening thought you want to "push it away," to stop thinking about it. But if you made yourself think it through again and again, pretty soon it would go from scary to boring. And then you might not have to think about it anymore at all!

The actual exposure to the content of the thoughts can be performed in any number of ways, such as writing a story describing the negative events actually happening and repeatedly reading the story aloud. Or recording a narration of the thoughts and listening to them for half an hour each day. Although such a direct confrontation with what is often extremely disturbing content can be difficult for both patient and therapist, it almost inevitably leads to rapid reductions in the level of affect that the thoughts are able to trigger and to a corresponding reduction in their frequency. In constructing the story (or other form of exposure) the therapist's task is to balance the degree of anxiety that the patient is currently willing to experience with the need to make the exercise effective by inviting as explicit content as possible. Although the form of the narrative can be directed by the therapist, most of the content should come directly from the patient, often in the form of answers to questions such as "What do you think would happen?" or "What would you be feeling if . . . ," and so on. This reliance on the patient for content ensures that the exposure does not do more than make deliberate what is already happening anyway without control. In other words, the patient who is already engaged in actively trying to avoid this content is not being introduced to new material that might be overly anxiety provoking or developmentally inappropriate.

Below is an example of a story constructed with a 17-year-old boy who had an obsessive fear of losing the key to his home and causing it to be broken into. As a consequence of his obsession the young man had taken to engaging in ritualized searching for his key each and every time he left a room or got out of the car.

> You're walking home from school when you think you hear a little clink, the sound of something metallic falling. You want to stop and check if you dropped your key but you remind yourself that this is merely your OCD and so you keep walking without checking. But it was your key. You lost it and soon a bad person found the key. That night he came to your home. He opened the door and began collecting things he wanted to steal. Your father wakes up and confronts him, and the burglar shoots him dead. Your mother tries to call the police but the burglar sees her and kills her, too. You're at your parents' funeral. You are standing there crying and your sister is there crying and saying "This is all your fault. If only you had checked that it wasn't your key this never would have happened. You killed them."

This scenario, which is abbreviated from the one used in treatment, was clearly distressing to the patient the first time he heard it. However, with repetition even the impact of an unpleasant story becomes dulled. Although constantly avoiding the thought increases the level of anxiety it provokes, systematic exposure rapidly reduces the effect of listening to the content. This particular scenario also exemplifies another aspect of cognitive exposure that is beneficial in many cases. For many individuals with anxious thoughts who fear catastrophic events, the fear of personal responsibility for the event can be as frightening as the fear of the actual event happening. Imagining berating oneself for having caused a catastrophe can be as distressing as imagining the catastrophe itself. In OCD this fear can be a significant contributor to the drive to complete the rituals or to undo the distressing thought. In the story above, this facet of avoidance (avoiding responsibility for the outcome) is addressed by including the phrase: *You want to stop and check if you dropped your key but you remind yourself that this is merely your OCD and so you keep walking without checking.* This includes a direct exposure to the personal responsibility and the fear of becoming culpable by resisting the OCD. The responsibility is highlighted again in the description of the sister accusing the patient of causing the parents' death through his actions.

PARENT GUIDANCE

Working closely with the parents is a key ingredient in achieving successful exposure work, especially for those exposures that are done at home or in the absence of the therapist.

Parent Involvement

Ensuring that a parent is aware of the behavioral tasks a child is supposed to complete in a given week will usually increase the likelihood of the behaviors occurring. This should not be confused with making the parents responsible for the completion of the homework. In most cases it is wise to specifically caution the parent against "making children" do the exposures as this will probably serve to solidify the view that the exposures are something the parents want done rather than something the children are undertaking for their own goals. Instead, parents should support the process by reminding children, helping them to make time for the exposures, and, when necessary, filling their own part, as in the case of children with separation anxiety whose parents leave the home for the exposure.

Emphasize the Gradual Nature of Exposures

The desire to see one's child doing better, the impact of the anxiety on the family life, and the fear of a long and interminable therapeutic process can all combine to make parents anxious to proceed rapidly through the exposure hierarchy. Counteracting this urge is an important part of the parent work for the therapist. In our work with parents of anxious children we often repeat the mantra that "the longer route is almost always the shorter one"; in other words, a gradual, cautious, and restrained pace leads to quicker results and improvements than an attempt to charge ahead and make rapid gains.

For many children the first steps on the exposure hierarchy actually are something that children are likely to do occasionally anyway. For example, a child with a severe dog phobia might rate "walking with mommy through a park" as anxiety provoking, although this is something the child may occasionally do without argument. Choosing an initial step that the child sometimes does in any event is a good way of ensuring success in this early stage and increasing motivation for further exposures. Consequentially, it is misguided to discount this exposure as being "less real" for the fact that it happens sometimes without treatment. In fact, just because a child sometimes does something on occasion is not proof that this does not cause some anxiety. Most children regularly engage in activities that cause them some degree of fear. Additionally, by choosing to focus on the situation in the form of a planned exposure, the child's anxiety is usually heightened and a situation that might usually cause only minor anxiety can create significant discomfort. The conclusion is—don't rush it! No exposure is too easy to start with!

Gradual Generalization

The following scenario is familiar to anyone engaged in work with families of anxious children: A child who has been avoiding a situation for some time, for example, a child who has refused to eat milk products because of a fear of spoiled food, completes an exposure in which he or she eats cottage cheese, perhaps even one day past the expiration date.

That night at dinner the family has cheese and the child refuses to eat perfectly fresh cottage cheese. The parents may feel exasperated because "After all, you just did this today!"

Generalizing the lessons learned through exposure is a necessary process and one that almost always will occur, but it is not instantaneous. The fact that children managed, through commitment to a treatment plan and by focusing their will and determination, to overcome a difficult experience, does not automatically make them willing or prepared to overcome every similar experience in day-to-day life. This is not a stubborn clinging to pathology or anxiety but rather an intermediate step that children will work through gradually at their own individual pace. Parents who miss this point and expect a child to be able to apply the exposure paradigm to all other situations will lower a child's willingness to proceed with more exposures. Children will come to realize that the implication of doing exposures will be an expectation to do the same all the time and they will resist making more progress.

Reframe "Failed Exposures"

Dana was 10 years old and terrified to walk to school alone. She was in the fourth grade and school was just down the block with no streets to cross, but she refused to make the 3-minute walk by herself. She tried it during the first week of school and had been flooded by scary thoughts about everything from monsters in the bushes to her mother disappearing while she was on the way. She was used to being in school alone but the walk there was just too hard. In treatment Dana and her parents had worked out a plan to address this. Dana would walk to school by herself and her mother would watch her all the way from the window. The next day Dana set out and her mother stood at the window to watch her. The mother observed as Dana began the walk confidently, her head up and her back straight. Soon, though, her posture changed. She seemed to become less sure of herself and about a third of the way to school she stopped and hesitated. Slowly, she took a few more faltering steps and when she was almost half of the way to school, she turned around and ran back home. When she got into the house Dana was crying: "I can't do it," she blurted out, "I'm too frightened."

Dana's mother was faced with a serious dilemma: How is she to respond to Dana's failure to live up to the plan and walk to school alone? She was disappointed and frustrated and could the feel the words forming in her mouth: "You were half way there—you could just as easily have run to school rather than home," she wanted to say; "We made a plan and I did my part—why couldn't you do yours?"

Saying those things seems natural but they would only serve to confirm to Dana what she already suspected—that she is weak, helpless, and something of a nuisance. Perhaps even a disappointment to her mom. Seeing things in that light would also mask an important facet of the morning's experiment—*She had walked halfway to school alone!* That was actually a tremendous accomplishment that stood the risk of being lost in the disappointment of not having gone all the way. Helping parents to reframe a partial success as what it actually is—a win rather than a loss—is an important part of parent guidance for anxious children.

In therapy, when a child is unable to follow through with a planned exposure, most good therapists will take the responsibility on themselves rather than laying it on the child: "I guess I really miscalculated with that one—I don't know what I was thinking." Or perhaps, "Wow, I'm amazed you got that much of it done—I felt like I had really pushed too far and I can't believe you did that well." By highlighting the partial success rather than focusing on the empty half of the glass, and taking explicit responsibility for overassessing the child's current capacity, a sense of accomplishment can be restored and motivation can be maintained.

For some parents, understanding just how difficult an exposure might be for the child is difficult. Therapists who regularly work with anxiety-disordered patients are used to seeing the exposures through their patients' eyes and have usually gained an appreciation for how challenging they can be. For parents, to whom the exposure might seem like doing an everyday thing that should come naturally, this can be harder. Helping parents to adopt the child's perspective is vital to their ability to interact supportively with the child. Sometimes asking parents to imagine that they were the ones doing something that would be hard for them is a start.

The father of a young girl with OCD was frustrated by the "evasive tactics" she would employ to avoid doing the exposures the therapist had suggested as homework. She said she wanted to get better but she always had an excuse to procrastinate. Her father was growing more and more irritated and the homework time became increasingly stressful for both of them. I asked the father to imagine that he was in the position of having to do something utterly repulsive to him because it was the only way to get better. "Imagine that, in order to overcome a problem that's been bothering you—you had to eat one cup of earthworms every evening. Your doctor is standing there holding out this cup of slimy, disgusting worms and telling you to hurry up already—it's the only way to get better. Wouldn't you try every excuse to delay? Wouldn't you use every evasive tactic imaginable? Instead of being angry about the procrastination, try to recognize what an accomplishment it is to be trying to do this at all. For someone with an anxiety disorder, exposures are hard." That father summed it up as succinctly as I've ever heard it put: "Yes," he said. "It's F*ing hard!"

PROGRAM FOR BEDTIME-RELATED SEPARATION ANXIETY—THE YALE PLAN FOR GETTING YOUR KID TO SLEEP IN HIS OWN BED

Many children experience separation anxiety, particularly around bedtime. In fact, in our experience, not being able to sleep in their own bed is one of the most common complaints among parents of anxious children. The principles of gradual repeated exposures can be applied to this common complaint very successfully. Many therapists advise parents to create a gradual process by slowly increasing the distance from the parents' bed. In this plan, children are first moved to a mattress alongside the parents' bed and then the mattress is gradually inched away toward the children's room until they are back in their own room, when they move into their own bed.

In our experience, there is a better approach. We advise inviting the child to play a game that we could call "making believe you are going to sleep in your bed." Children are encouraged to put on a kind of show, tricking an imaginary audience into thinking they are going to sleep in their own bed, although they actually know this is not going to be the case.

To do this, the first stage is often making sure that the child actually has a bed to sleep in. Many children will not have slept in their bed for so long that it has been turned into a "closet," been transferred to a sibling for them to sleep in, or, in one case, actually removed from the room. The child can think of this as setting the stage, or preparing the necessary props for the show. The bed is made up completely including sheets and blankets and made ready as if the child were to sleep there that night.

Next, children will go through the motions of going to bed. They will prepare for sleep, including washing up, putting on PJs, and so on, and will then get into their bed—for a predetermined length of time. Ideally, children will be actively involved in setting the length of time they will be in bed. For many children the first stage in this process will be only a minute or so long. Children know full well that after that minute is over the parents will come to let them know that the time is up, and they will then move into their bed for the rest of the night. As long as children have completed the prescribed amount of time in bed—they have successfully completed their task and are welcome back in the parents' bed without further demands.

It is important that parents not try to encourage the child to stay longer than was planned. So even if children appear perfectly comfortable after the time is up, we advise parents not to suggest that they "just stay there." Rather, they should explicitly invite the children to their room and praise them for completing their assignment. After repeating a given length of time for two or three nights, the time can be gradually lengthened in small increments. Usually by the time the duration reaches 10 to 15 minutes, children will have fallen asleep in their own bed—in which case the parents leave them there for the rest of the night and in the morning celebrate their success at sleeping in bed. Nevertheless, even after a child has stayed the entire night, the plan continues unaltered the following night and so forth until sleeping in bed has become a regular and consistent occurrence.

This plan has had extremely high rates of success with parents, including those whose children had slept with them for many years. The secret lies in the fact that by predefining the amount of time a child will lay in bed, a situation is created in which the child is in bed but is not anxious. This is because they know it is only for a limited amount of time. The natural consequence of lying in bed when not particularly anxious is falling asleep. Children could lie awake for much more than 15 minutes if they think they need to be in bed alone all night and could even keep themselves (and their parents) up by calling to the parents or crying. But by assuring the child that this is only a "game" for a set and brief amount of time, the anxiety is eliminated and the child forms a new association between being in bed and feelings of calm and relaxation.

For children who have trouble both going to sleep and waking up during the night, we recommend tackling bedtime first, before trying to get children to stay in bed when they wake up at night. If children are unable to go to sleep at bedtime they are probably equally, or even more, unable to stay in bed after waking up because they have no experience of falling asleep in bed. Only after children are falling asleep alone in bed should parents apply the same principles to middle of the nights waking—by encouraging children to stay in bed for a fixed amount of time before coming in to the parents' room and by supplying them with a way of measuring that time. For example, a music player preset with a song of a specific duration could be placed near the bed and the child asked to listen one time to the entire song before moving to the parents' room.

REFERENCES

Dymond, S., & Roche, B. (2009). A contemporary behavior analysis of anxiety and avoidance. [Peer Reviewed]. *Behavior Analyst, 32*(1), 7–27.

Eun-Jung, K. (2005). The effect of the decreased safety behaviors on anxiety and negative thoughts in social phobics. *Journal of Anxiety Disorders, 19*(1), 69–86. doi:10.1016/j.janxdis.2003.11.002

Hofmann, S. G., Sawyer, A. T., Witt, A. A., & Oh, D. (2010). The effect of mindfulness-based therapy on anxiety and depression: A meta-analytic review. *Journal of Consulting and Clinical Psychology, 78*(2), 169–183. doi:10.1037/a0018555

Lebowitz, E. R., Vitulano, L. A., Mataix-Cols, D., & Leckman, J. (2011). Editorial perspective: When OCD takes over . . . the family! Coercive and disruptive behaviours in paediatric obsessive compulsive disorder. *Journal of Child Psychology and Psychiatry, 52*(12), 1249–1250.

Lissek, S., Powers, A. S., McClure, E. B., Phelps, E. A., Woldeha-wariat, G., Grillon, C., & Pine, D. S. (2005). Classical fear conditioning in the anxiety disorders: A meta-analysis. *Behaviour Research and Therapy, 43*(11), 1391–1424.

Logue, A. W. (1985). Conditioned food aversion learning in humans. *Annals of the New York Academy of Sciences, 443,* 316–329.

Logue, A. W., Ophir, I., & Strauss, K. E. (1981). The acquisition of taste aversions in humans. *Behaviour Research and Therapy, 19*(4), 319–333.

Moulding, R., & Kyrios, M. (2006). Anxiety disorders and control related beliefs: The exemplar of obsessive-compulsive disorder (OCD). *Clinical Psychology Review, 26*(5), 573–583.

Pervin, L. A. (1963). The need to predict and control under conditions of threat. *Journal of Personality, 31,* 570–587.

Rescorla, R. A. (1988). Pavlovian conditioning. It's not what you think it is. *American Psychologist, 43*(3), 151–160.

Salkovskis, P. M., Clark, D. M., Hackmann, A., Wells, A., & Gelder, M. G. (1999). An experimental investigation of the role of safety-seeking behaviours in the maintenance of panic disorder with agoraphobia. *Behaviour Research and Therapy, 37*(6), 559–574.

Thwaites, R., & Freeston, M. H. (2005). Safety-seeking behaviours: Fact or function? How can we clinically differentiate between safety behaviours and adaptive coping strategies across anxiety disorders? *Behavioural and Cognitive Psychotherapy, 33*(02), 177–188. doi:10.1017/S1352465804001985

Waltz, T. J., & Hayes, S. C. (2010). *Acceptance and commitment therapy: cognitive and behavioral theories in clinical practice* (pp. 148–192). New York, NY: Guilford Press.

Weems, C. F., Silverman, W. K., Rapee, R. M., & Pina, A. A. (2003). The role of control in childhood anxiety disorders. *Cognitive Therapy and Research, 27*(5), 557–568. doi:10.1023/a:1026307121386

Wells, A., Clark, D. M., Salkovskis, P., Ludgate, J., Hackmann, A., & Gelder, M. (1995). Social phobia: The role of in-situation safety behaviors in maintaining anxiety and negative beliefs. *Behavior Therapy, 26*(1), 153–161. doi:10.1016/s0005-7894(05)80088-7

CHAPTER SIX

Physiological Tools for Treating Anxiety

Anxiety affects the body in powerful ways in both the short and long term. For some children, fear of the physical manifestations of anxiety is the major component in the anxiety disorder. Teaching a child tools to "take back control" of the body can help restore confidence and build coping strategies.

Key points in this chapter:

- Experiencing anxiety involves a cascade of physiological changes that can be distressing.
- Physiological elements of anxiety include both acute and chronic effects.
- Relaxation skills can help a child regulate anxiety and reduce the fear of anxious arousal.
- Parents can model less fearful attitudes toward the physical elements of anxiety and the use of relaxation.

THE PHYSICAL ELEMENT OF ANXIETY

The physical aspect of the alarm response is an important element in the manifestation of anxiety and its treatment. The cascade of physiological reactions that take place when a child's anxiety system is triggered can probably be thought of as the most basic of all the components of the reaction. Indeed, the physiological changes seen in humans experiencing alarm resemble in many ways those witnessed in many other species, and have their roots in a more ancient evolutionary period than our more "modern" cognitions.

It is helpful to subdivide the physical aspects of anxiety into two main categories based on the time frame in which they occur and the toll they take on those who experience them.

Acute Physical Response

The acute physical response can be thought of as all those bodily changes that make up what is often termed the *flight or fight* reaction. Some of the more readily noticeable shifts in the way one's body works or feels can include increased heart rate, trembling, shallow breathing, sweating, and many others. Some of the less immediately obvious changes can include things like feeling coldness in the hands or feet, dry mouth, and some changes that are too subtle to ever be noticed by the person experiencing the anxiety, such as pupil dilation. One theory of panic attacks attributes them to misinterpretation of body cues as signs of imminent suffocation (Klein, 1993). This approach has garnered empirical support from studies in which subjects are exposed to carbon dioxide (CO_2), which mimics suffocation. Anxious children responded to the experience with more panic-like symptoms than children not suffering from anxiety disorders (Pine et al., 1998). Conversely, children diagnosed with congenital central hypoventilation syndrome, a disease that makes them unable to detect elevated rates of CO_2 or to hyper-ventilate as a result of it, were found to manifest fewer anxiety disorders than others. These findings contribute to the view that one risk for the development of anxiety disorders is a focus on physiological arousal and misinterpretation of it as dangerous. For children suffering from anxiety disorders, the focus on internal cues such as elevated heart rate or rapid breathing creates a self-reinforcing loop, a kind of vicious cycle where any sign of anxiety triggers arousal and the interpretation of the arousal increases the anxiety.

In fact, a physically healthy child is not at immediate risk from the experience of acute or repeated anxiety. A healthy person is fully capable of enduring anxiety without any short-term ill effects. Healthy children do not have heart attacks because they become anxious or suffer collapses because of feeling afraid. In working with both children and parents, stressing this point is crucial. If a child believes that there is real danger in becoming anxious for even a short time, then it becomes imperative to do everything possible to avoid such experiences. If parents believe that anxiety will truly harm their child, then they will inevitably be compelled to protect them from anxiety.

> Some time ago I had the misfortune of needing to undergo a root canal that took considerable time and was quite a challenge to both myself and the dentist who performed it. I had a lot of confidence in my doctor who is a skilled and gentle man but found myself being somewhat irritated by him throughout the procedure. Whenever he needed to ask me if a certain spot was sensitive or not he would say "Do you feel any discomfort here? How about here, any discomfort?" I felt like yelling at him: "Discomfort? No, no discomfort—what I feel is *pain*!" It was only after he had finished the procedure that I realized that, although he might have hurt my feelings in the process, he had actually saved me quite a bit of pain. By insisting on defining my experience as one of discomfort, he had helped me to gradually come to experience it more along those lines as well.

The best description for experiences of acute anxiety, in situations that are not actually life threatening such as real traffic accidents, natural disasters, or the like, is one of *discomfort*. Although children may feel that this term does not capture the full phenomenological scope of the situation or that it belittles their anguish, framing the experience as discomfort can allow the adult to maintain a realistic and supportive attitude. Acting as though the feelings are actually catastrophic may be more in line with the child's inner beliefs at the time, but can only serve to reinforce his or her belief that anxiety must be avoided at all costs.

Chronic Physical Stress

Although the immediate and acute fear response inevitably subsides within a short time from when it is triggered, there are physical effects caused by the recurring activation of the alarm system and the persistent hypervigilance typical of individuals with anxiety disorders. Some of the more common complaints can include various aches and pains such as headache, stomachache, or back pain, tiredness and lack of energy, or symptoms such as gastrointestinal upset (Campo et al., 2004; Dufton, Dunn, & Compas, 2009; McWilliams, Cox, & Enns, 2003). These may be caused directly by the overactivation of the sympathetic system or indirectly through sleep deprivation, irregular eating, sedentariness, and inactivity or other effects on the child's habits and schedule.

There is significant research pointing to the deleterious effects of anxiety-related chronic stress on health, immune response, mood, and other elements of day-to-day life (Brosschot, Gerin, & Thayer, 2006). The hypothalamic-pituitary-adrenal axis is the hormonal system charged with regulating stress, and persistent activation of this complex system can cause many of the functions necessary for healthy and adaptive behavior to become unregulated (Kallen et al., 2008). Although to many families and practitioners these symptoms may appear less significant than the more dramatic indications of acute stress, their importance for the child's health may actually be considerably greater.

Next we discuss a number of skills that can be helpful in mitigating or alleviating the negative physiological aspects of anxiety.

Relaxation

Relaxation training is probably one of the most polarizing of all anxiety management skills. Some therapists swear by the importance of teaching anxious children to relax their bodies and would never consider treating anxiety without addressing this basic skill. Others feel it is over-emphasized and is really more of a placebo than a treatment. Among patients, opinions are similarly divided. There are many children who use relaxation exercises to great effect and feel that learning the skill provides them with a sense of control over a body that for much of the time was "running away from them" with uncontrollable anxiety symptoms. Other children feel bored and unaffected by the techniques. For some, the attempts at deliberate relaxation actually seem to para-doxically raise anxiety levels, as though lowering their defenses triggers alarms that replace calmness with increased vigilance. Our own attitude toward these skills echoes what we have stated for all of the techniques discussed in this book. Namely, they work best for those for whom they work! By offering a child a metaphoric buffet of skills, introducing all but insisting on no particular one approach or program, a child can be free to experiment. When relaxation is effective and is presented as a skill for the child rather than a chore to be completed, it can be adopted with enthusiasm. For children who have been tense and rigid for so long that they have stopped being aware of the tension itself, the relief that comes with being able to lower the strain can be akin to putting down a heavy load one has carried for so long that it has almost become unnoticed.

Below are two suggested texts for teaching relaxation. The first, targeting both muscle relaxation and breathing, is aimed at relaxation training to be practiced in nonstressful situations until a degree of proficiency is attained and then gradually brought to bear on anxiety-provoking moments. It requires a degree of persistence to achieve this level of competence and the therapist is advised to avoid making this practice into a homework-like assignment that will antagonize the child. For example, it is likely that most of the learning actually occurs within the first 5 minutes or so of each practice session. Demanding that a child engage in much longer sessions is likely to breed defiance while earning steeply diminishing returns. Additionally, many children find the kind of introspective meditation that is generally associated with relaxation exercises exceedingly boring. For some, mindful self-reflection is soothing, but for many it is closer to torture and we advise openness to activities that a child can engage in while practicing relaxation training such as listening to music or a story, watching a favorite (albeit not too stimulating) show on TV, or stroking a pet.

1. Take a moment to just notice the way you are right now. Are you sitting down? Lying down perhaps? Can you feel the surface of whatever is supporting you? If you are not comfortable, change your position a little; there's no right way to do this. Let's take a tour of your body and try to help it relax a little as we go. You're completely in control of your body and can make it do wonderful things. You can make your hands, feet, or fingers do anything you want. Right now you're going to make it relax. Another time you could experiment with making your body walk, or jump really high; right now let's get it to really relax. We can start from your

feet. They work really hard all day. They carry you around all the time. They'd probably love to rest a little. Let them rest a bit. Let your feet choose the angle they want from your leg. Don't hold them, just let them drop however they want. I bet your feet appreciate the attention. Your legs would love to relax as well. You have lots of muscles in your legs. There are muscles in your calves, your knees, your thighs. Let them all take a little rest. Let your legs just lie there for a bit held by your chair or bed. You don't need to hold yourself up right now, you can let yourself be supported and rest. Your stomach can be soft or hard. When it's hard, it is working. It is being strong. Right now it can be soft. Feel your belly relaxing. Let your back just be supported as well. Your shoulders are also always working hard. They keep you upright. And they hold you stiff and steady. Right now they can slump a little. Let them fall a little and your neck can relax as well. Even your face has lots of muscles. Your mouth, your jaw, they're very strong. Now they can also rest. Your mouth can be a little open. It doesn't matter. It's okay now. If your chin wants to fall a little toward your chest, that's fine. Let your forehead relax. Even your scalp can loosen up a little. Your whole body can rest for a bit. Now is a good time for that. And when your body is relaxed, you may notice that your breathing changes a little, too. It may go a little slower. The muscles inside you also want to rest. Your lungs need some rest. Now is the right time for that. Let your breathing slow. You can help by breathing in slowly through your nose. Your lungs really like that. It fills them with clean relaxing air. You can breathe out slowly as well. If you feel like it you can breathe out through your mouth. That's very calming. It tells your whole body that everything is fine. Just keep breathing like that while your body rests for a bit. It will thank you later. It will be strong when you need it to be; right now it's resting. Just resting for a bit.

The second text (below) is aimed at different situations and, in some cases, at different children as well. This exercise is most useful for times of acute stress or for children who find relaxation to be anxiety inducing rather than relieving. One of the authors of this text remembers when, as a teenager, his mother acquired a recording that contained the supposedly soothing sounds of whales singing in the ocean. The sound was so aggravating that within very little time he threatened to break the record if he had to listen to it one more time!

Some of the paradoxically anxiety-increasing responses to relaxation may stem, as mentioned, from a reluctance to lower vigilance levels, and this is particularly true in times of acute alarm (Moulding & Kyrios, 2006). The very act of relaxation flies directly in the face of the natural instinct to overcome threat. Keep in mind that anxiety in the context of an anxiety disorder is mostly identical to healthy anxiety in the context of a real threat. Not surprisingly, there is little natural inclination toward relaxation in those circumstances. In fact, attempts by others to induce relaxation when a child is feeling frightened or aroused can lead not only to resistance and increased anxiety but also to hostility and aggressive behavior.

> Imagine that your child was late coming home one day, not answering the phone, and you didn't know where she was. You might be flooded with terrible thoughts about things that could have happened or places she might be. Now imagine that I came over, stood next to you, and in a silky soothing voice said softly: "Now I want you to relax, just breathe deeply." You'd probably not appreciate my attempt at relaxation and might be really angry. You might want to yell "Don't tell me to relax—my kid is missing!" A scared child will often react in much the same way. Relaxation, in the face of what feels like danger, can be very counterintuitive and provoke anger.

An additional consideration is that in advising children to relax, take control of their body, and regulate their feelings, we are unwittingly setting up a situation in which any remaining anxiety signifies their failure to comply with this advice. Despite the therapist's best intentions, telling children to relax is often the same as telling them that they can do so and that if they feel they cannot then either their anxiety is particularly great or they are inadequate. Neither conclusion is one that will serve to reduce anxiety. For these reasons it is often more helpful to take a more roundabout route to relaxation without actually asking a child to relax at all. The text below is an example of such a technique.

2. Now I'm going to count to three. When I get to three, I want you to tighten and squeeze all the muscles in your body, as if you're turning into a really tightly wound spring. You should make your hands into really hard fists. Imagine your fingers turning white from the pressure; pull your arms in tight and stiffen them, close your eyes tight, scrunch up your face and bite down as hard as you can; hold your stomach in and make it really hard; stiffen your legs from hip to heel, as if they were turning into iron rods. Your whole body is going to be totally taut when I count to three. Okay: one, two, and three! Now! Clench your fists, your arms, eyes, lips, teeth, stomach and legs! Good! Hold it like that. Now I'm going to count to 20, and when I get to 20, you can let everything go.[1]

This small exercise is particularly helpful because it not only restores a sense of control it also reduces the child's fear of the anxiety response itself. By simulating a body in extreme anxiety it creates an impromptu exposure of the sensations of the acute anxious response and gradually desensitizes the child to them. In addition, by not directing the child to reduce anxiety, feel calm, or otherwise relax, both of the risks mentioned earlier are mitigated. A child cannot feel a sense of failure at not relaxing because that was never the explicit goal. The sense of swimming upstream and trying to take the body in the opposite direction of the one it is striving for is also removed by engaging in deliberate tension rather than relaxation.

Healthy Living

Another way to counteract the physiological effects of anxiety is to promote healthy habits in the anxious child.

---

[1]A variation of this exercise includes directing children to breathe rapid shallow breaths during the time they are clenched and then to breathe normally. This is helpful in simulating anxiety and reducing the fear of anxious symptoms but can cause some children to experience dizziness or nausea.

I once worked with a man who came to treatment because he constantly felt anxious and restless. He attributed his symptoms to the stress of his job and the anxiety he felt about his financial situation. He complained that he was always worrying and never felt relaxed. Before beginning treatment I asked him to describe what a typical day looked like for him. It turned out he went to bed very late because he liked to play online gambling games, though he would only play for "make-believe money," not actually gambling. He would then have to get up a few hours later and he used extraordinary amounts of coffee to get through the day because he was so tired. I tried to help him see that even the best treatment in the world would have a difficult challenge helping a man to relax when he was running on caffeine and little sleep.

Most children, young ones in particular, will probably not be drinking inordinate amounts of coffee, but unhealthy habits can undermine even the best treatment for anxiety.

Sleep
Sleeping a reasonable number of hours a night is of real importance to how one will feel during the day. However, as with the other habits we discuss, it is not only important to sleep enough—it is also important to sleep well. For instance, teenagers might sleep from 4 A.M. until 5 in the afternoon each day. That would result in 13 hours of sleep but they might not feel particularly well rested or healthy. Sleeping at night is more beneficial than sleeping during the day.

Eating
With food, too, it is not only important to eat enough but to eat well. This includes both the choice of food and the regularity with which it is eaten. We strongly recommend eating regular meals that are reasonably well-balanced. Although choosing organic vegetables over others may not make much difference in anxiety, eating generally healthy foods and staying away from caffeine (which comes in Coca-Cola as well as coffee) will. Another aspect of eating well is the social aspect of food. Eating alone in one's room every day, or doing it while on the run, will not promote as much well-being as sitting down to a meal with other people.

Exercise

Physical exercise is a wonderful counterbalance to anxiety, and incorporating a measure of physical activity into the day can reduce overall anxiety as well as leading to short-term bursts of confidence and well-being. For a child who is school phobic, for example, starting the day with a 20-minute walk might provide the necessary boost needed to summon up the courage to get to class. Overexercising can also be a problem, however, particularly when driven by low body image, and the activity should be monitored appropriately.

In general we recommend regular communication with the primary health-care provider and discussing the living habits in the context of the anxiety. Although some parents shy from discussing emotional problems with the pediatrician, this kind of communication can be an invaluable tool and asset. One way to explain to a child or parent the importance of habits for anxiety is to consider the way unhealthy habits might be interpreted by an anxious brain:

> Think about when people usually don't have enough food, or don't get enough sleep. If someone is not eating, what is more likely—that all is well in their life or that there is some problem in the environment? Usually if there is not enough food or sleep it is because something is seriously wrong. Perhaps a war is going on, or a famine. Over history people have probably always slept and eaten better in tranquil times when all was well. So if your body is not getting food or sleep or proper exercise, that could serve as a sign for your brain that you have a serious problem. What will that make you? More anxious!

PARENT GUIDANCE

Helping parents to become familiar with the relaxation techniques described earlier offers numerous advantages in treating a child with anxiety. Clearly the presence of an adult in the home who can coach in the practice of relaxation or remind the child to "tense up" when appropriate can be an aid in implementing the strategies outside of the doctor's office. In fact, many clinicians find the compliance rate with exercise regimens to be so low that without the parent's involvement the hope of a child actually practicing daily relaxation times seems vanishingly small. Nevertheless, the role that parents can play after they achieved some familiarity with the skills is not limited to that of coach or trainer.

A major contributor to the terror a child feels when anxiety spikes is related to a fear that those physical sensations will never subside. By tricking children into believing that avoiding the anxiety-provoking stimulus is the only avenue to ever feeling all right again and by compounding that belief with the idea that the body cannot sustain anxiety over time, the anxiety generates very catastrophic interpretations of the situation. Children often voice these beliefs plainly, as if stating the obvious: "I needed to get out of there or I'd explode!," "I couldn't handle it for another second," and "I almost died." That fear can only be exacerbated by the sight of parents frantic with worry and uncertainty. Reassurance seems hollow when it is provided by adults who have no confidence in their own words. Parents who are equipped with a plan for how they are to act are already helping their child just by exuding less helplessness and more confidence.

Role playing with parents with their own behavior when faced with a child's anxiety and helping them to become familiar with the words they will use under stress can lead to more productive behavior and less anxiety for everyone involved. Additionally, in the absence of any plan of action, most of us, parents and clinicians alike, will usually fall back on what we know best—talking. "What are you worried about now?"; "It is going to be okay." Such well-intentioned attempts at reassurance are all equally unlikely to succeed. Children in the throes of panic are just not receptive to verbal communication of the kind that is helpful in other situations. Alternatively, parents may feel they have no choice but to take action to protect the child and aid in avoiding the situation that creates the anxiety, a strategy more likely to succeed in the short-term but also one that inevitably leads to increased anxiety in the future.

REFERENCES

Brosschot, J. F., Gerin, W., & Thayer, J. F. (2006). The perseverative cognition hypothesis: A review of worry, prolonged stress-related physiological activation, and health. *Journal of Psychosomatic Research*, *60*(2), 113–124. doi:10.1016/j.jpsychores.2005.06.074

Campo, J. V., Bridge, J., Ehmann, M., Altman, S., Lucas, A., Birmaher, B., . . . Brent, D. A. (2004). Recurrent abdominal pain, anxiety, and depression in primary care. *Pediatrics, 113*(4), 817–824.

Dufton, L. M., Dunn, M. J., & Compas, B. E. (2009). Anxiety and somatic complaints in children with recurrent abdominal pain and anxiety disorders. *Journal of Pediatric Psychology, 34*(2), 176–186.

Kallen, V. L., Tulen, J. H. M., Utens, E. M. W. J., Treffers, P. D. A., De Jong, F. H., & Ferdinand, R. F. (2008). Associations between HPA axis functioning and level of anxiety in children and adolescents with an anxiety disorder. *Depression and Anxiety, 25*(2), 131–141. doi:10.1002/da.20287

Klein, D. F. (1993). False suffocation alarms, spontaneous panics, and related conditions. An integrative hypothesis. *Archives of General Psychiatry, 50*(4), 306–317.

McWilliams, L. A., Cox, B. J., & Enns, M. W. (2003). Mood and anxiety disorders associated with chronic pain: An examination in a nationally representative sample. *Pain, 106*(1–2), 127–133. doi:10.1016/s0304-3959(03)00301-4

Moulding, R., & Kyrios, M. (2006). Anxiety disorders and control related beliefs: The exemplar of obsessive-compulsive disorder (OCD). *Clinical Psychology Review, 26*(5), 573–583.

Pine, D. S., Coplan, J. D., Papp, L. A., Klein, R. G., Martinez, J. M., Kovalenko, P., . . . Gorman, J. M. (1998). Ventilatory physiology of children and adolescents with anxiety disorders. *Archives of General Psychiatry, 55*(2), 123–129.

CHAPTER SEVEN

Emotion-Based Tools for Treating Anxiety

The cognitive, physiological, and behavioral elements of anxiety are accompanied by an emotional component. Most often the feeling of fear accompanies anxiety but other emotions can also play a role. Learning skills to change or regulate the emotional experience is another way of coping with anxiety that many children naturally relate to.

Key points in this chapter:

- Anxiety can manifest with various emotions.
- Most often the emotion associated with anxiety is fear. Anxiety can also trigger emotions of anger, sadness, or unrest.
- Changing the emotion that accompanies a given situation can change the level of anxiety experienced.
- Many children relate very well to emotion-based skills and tools.
- Parents who can accept their child's emotional experience and model ways of coping will be better able to help their child overcome anxiety.

THE EMOTIONAL ELEMENT OF ANXIETY

The emotional impact of anxiety is the one we probably take most for granted. However, it is also the one that is usually least directly targeted for interventions. For many people anxiety is synonymous with *fear*, a word that describes its primary emotional component. Even when children are unable to voice any specific thoughts that trigger their anxiety or to describe the bodily changes that accompany it, they are usually aware of the *feelings* that go with being alarmed. In a manner that resembles that in which we described the physical manifestations of anxiety, the emotional component can also be divided into an acute and a more chronic phase.

Acute Emotional Response

The primary emotion associated with anxiety is fear. Emotions are difficult to describe, and an attempt to completely separate the emotional aspect from the other components of anxiety is an impossible feat, but feeling afraid is one of those things we just recognize when they occur. However, fear is not the only emotion closely tied to the acute phase of anxiety. Perhaps because of the survival function of anxiety and its role in identifying threats and dispensing with them as swiftly as possible, another emotional shift during anxious arousal is the one toward anger and hostility.

Children experiencing anxiety are often described as being more angry or confrontational in their behavior, and the relationship between the two emotions has long been noted (Beck et al., 2005; Bowlby, 1969; Hewitt et al., 2002). Parents confronted by a child's oppositional behavior are often distraught at what they see as deterioration in their child's personality or character. For the therapist, children's anger can be considerably harder to contain than is their fear, as the therapist becomes a convenient target for children's ire. Correctly identifying a child's emotion as stemming from anxiety rather than an inherent anger or hostility toward the clinician can be important in assuming a supportive pose that will enable child and therapist to overcome the issue and forge a successful working alliance.

In Chapter 8 we discuss the importance of helping parents to form a supportive attitude toward a child suffering from anxiety. Support in the context of fearful emotions denotes an attitude, which conveys both acceptance of the emotion and a belief in the child's ability to overcome or withstand those feelings to at least some degree. By combining acceptance of children's experience with a confidence that they can behave differently nonetheless, support is accomplished. A similar principle can allow for successful management of anxiety-driven anger or hostility. Integrating an explicit acceptance of the anger children are feeling can go hand in hand with a belief in their ability to overcome that emotion to at least some degree. Therapists often become trapped by the sense that only after the hostility has been eliminated can the work of therapy begin. But this may cause children to feel that the sessions are focusing on the least important issue to them, and can cause frustration for both parties. Conversely, a therapist might feel that his or her authority is being challenged and be unable to frame the behavior in the context of an anxiety issue. This will likely lead to either a referral to another clinician or to an arm wrestling–like contest that does little to improve the child's symptoms. A supportive stance will explicitly declare the therapist's acknowledgment of the child's experience and frame it as part of the anxious symptomatology. This is accompanied by nonconfrontational yet determined statements regarding the minimal conditions necessary for the therapy to continue. Here is an example of such a statement made to an 11-year-old child:

> Mark, I've been thinking since our last meeting and I want to tell you what I think. I understand that you feel a lot of anger toward me. You made it clear when we last spoke that you don't enjoy talking to me and that you feel pretty bad about being here at all. I want you to know that I get that and that it's okay for you to feel that way. The truth is just being anxious, nervous, or worried can make anyone much more upset at other people and it's natural to feel that way. I also think that you can act differently. Just letting yourself be angry is actually letting your feelings get in the way of you getting better. I am not angry at you but in order to help you we need to have some rules. The first is you can feel anything toward me and you can always tell me how you feel. The second rule is to talk respectfully to each other. That's really important. The last rule is: Even when anxiety makes you really angry we are going to not let that stop us from making you better.

Although no statement can ever ensure that a child will overcome anger or frustration to work with the therapist, adopting an attitude of support can lay the groundwork necessary to maximize the potential for fruitful collaboration. For situations in which working directly with the child is constantly or temporarily untenable, we devote a separate section in this book to parent guidance in the absence of child collaboration.

Chronic Emotional Response

As in the case of physiological features of anxiety, in the realm of emotion, too, the chronic effects of prolonged, recurrent, or pervasive anxiety can be more deleterious than the more dramatic yet short-lived elements of the acute phase. In considering the chronic emotional effects of anxiety it is probably just as productive to think about the emotions *not* being experienced because of anxiety rather than those that are actively present. Feeling afraid for much of the time is an immense emotional strain, and irritability, anger, or helplessness all negatively impact well-being. But being anxious can also dictate what you are *not*. For many children, chronic anxiety of the kind typical of an anxiety disorder will mean *not* being happy, *not* being interested in new things or experiences, *not* being motivated to achieve goals that are not directly related to the anxiety, or *not* being willing to risk social interaction (Kashdan, 2007). It is not surprising that just having any anxiety disorder is a significant risk factor for also developing a mood disorder like depression (Anderson & Hope, 2008; Dobson, 1985). Combined with a sense of helplessness and the lack of faith that the situation is likely to change for the better, these symptoms can cause significant impairment in a child, over and above the direct effects of anxiety such as avoidance of feared situations and stimuli.

> At first he wouldn't go anywhere unless I promised to stay with him the whole time. He would make me swear to it. But now he won't go at all, even if I beg him. He says it's not really fun and he'd rather just stay home. He says it's just not worth it.

An additional emotion-related aspect of persistent anxiety is the negative effect that it can have on a child's self-image and self-esteem. Consistently feeling weaker or less capable than others can lead children to view themselves less positively, as can the sensation of being "strange" and different (Kirkcaldy, Eysenck, Furnham, & Siefen, 1998). Children are typically unaware of how common a phenomenon anxiety actually is and may feel as though they alone experience the kind of problems they face. For this reason, helping a child to overcome a specific fear is not an ambitious enough goal in the treatment of pediatric anxiety. An additional goal should be providing the child with a higher tolerance for anxiety and an increased sense of competence and mastery. Without a doubt, the impact of such a shift on children's self-esteem is a great boon to their emotional well-being.

Using Other Emotions

It is challenging for a child to experience more than one conflicting or contradictory emotion at the same time. Although this is likely often a significant part of the problem in anxiety disorders, as it becomes harder to experience positive emotion alongside anxiety, it also offers a strategy to changing a child's inner state. If indeed one cannot feel two different things at once, then by evoking an emotion that is not part of the anxious repertoire, a child can deliberately steer his experience in a nonanxious direction. In fact, this works surprisingly well for many children. One way of explaining this to children can be to call to mind other situations in which this technique is used:

> Have you ever seen a movie in which two armies are pitched for battle and soldiers are just about to face off? Think about the officer and what he might be doing. Imagine him parading in front of the soldiers on his horse. He is talking to them about glory, about patriotic pride, about the anger they should feel toward the other side. He talks about their love for their homeland. These are all ways of stirring up powerful emotions — pride, anger, devotion to their land and their companions. As these emotions swell, the soldiers become less afraid and charge into battle without feelings of fear holding them back.

One emotion that can be particularly helpful for accomplishing this with a fearful child is that of humor or mirth. Simply choosing to feel *happy* instead of fearful usually is not realistic, but by causing a situation to take on a humorous or even absurd connotation, anxiety can be greatly reduced. A favorite application of this principle is found (as are many other psychological insights) in the *Harry Potter* series. In a class on defending themselves from the "Dark Arts" Harry and his mates learn to overcome the terror caused by a magical creature—the boggart. A boggart is a metaphor for anxiety itself—not actually having the power to harm a person directly but rather, magically taking on the form of whatever that person fears the most and filling them with paralyzing terror. The trick to overcoming a boggart is in eliciting humor rather than fear:

> The charm that repels a Boggart is simple, yet it requires force of mind. You see, the thing that really finishes a Boggart is laughter. What you need to do is force it to assume a shape that you find amusing. (Rowling, 1999)

The principle works equally well for the boggarts of our ("muggle") world. By conjuring up humor, either by imagining the feared stimulus in a funny form or by focusing on an unrelated funny thing such as a joke or a movie, anxiety can be diminished greatly.

> A girl of 9 was in treatment because of very persistent and extreme worry that her father would meet with a car accident during the day. The father worked as a salesman and spent a lot of time on the road, triggering her anxiety. She was constantly flooded with images of her father in a mangled vehicle, being removed from the scene by medics, or on life support in a hospital. With some encouragement she was persuaded to draw these scenes on paper and they were indeed quite horrific. After discussing the use of humor, an impish smile began to appear on her face. She took one of the pictures she had drawn and began to embellish it. Soon the intravenous tubes leading into her father were filled with chocolate milk, the monitor he was connected to was showing a smiley, and the nurse was putting a piece of spaghetti in his mouth instead of a thermometer. In another session she giggled as she transformed the scene of her father's accident into a movie set. As medics step forward to lift him from the wrecked car, a director steps forward and a speech bubble shows him yelling "Cut! Not enough blood! We have to film this all over again!"

For many children, however, humor seems so remotely detached from their experience that any attempt at mirth feels blithe or inappropriate.

It is useful to remember that although positive emotions are naturally preferable to negative ones, it will often be easier to replace fear with a competing emotion such as anger rather than a more pleasant sensation. When the anger is channeled appropriately, this can be a useful technique.

One particularly helpful strategy can be to direct the anger at the fear itself. Younger children can create a figure, perhaps a picture, sock puppet, or some other form, and then focus their anger and frustration on the representation. In this way anxiety is externalized, children are given the opportunity for some "payback" against their inner tormentor, and most important of all, fear subsides as the powerful emotion of rage takes its place. After some minutes tearing, throwing, hitting, or yelling at the anxiety doll, a child is almost certain to feel less afraid.

Holly was 9 and suffering from significant obsessive-compulsive disorder. She was tormented by near-constant thoughts about all the catastrophes that could occur to her family, particularly in storms or other natural phenomena. To alleviate some of the distress that these images evoked and to persuade herself that the scenarios would not be realized, she felt compelled to perform a variety of rituals that interfered with her and her family's day-to-day life. In treatment Holly was very brave; standing up to her fears and not allowing anxiety to be the bully who would push her around and make her do things against her will. Holly created a sock puppet of "Biff the bully" who represented her anxiety. She would punish him severely when anxiety reared its head. Standing up to Biff became a recurrent theme in her therapy, and channeling her anger in this way proved a successful strategy.

PARENT GUIDANCE

Through supportive actions and by refraining from behaviors that convey either overprotection or a negation of the child's inner feelings, parents can navigate the tricky waters of an anxious child's emotional challenges. Clinicians working with parents of children with anxiety all too often fall into a trap when a parent asks "But how can I help him feel differently?" This is the parent's greatest hope. It would indeed be wonderful if therapists could teach parents what to say so as to mold their children's feelings or shape them in more positive ways. Unfortunately, by attempting to provide parents with such magic words, the therapist is actually conveying the message that this is the parents' role. It is not! Given that even skilled therapists will not often be able to just make children feel differently, it would be surprising if they knew how to train parents to do so. This is unrealistic. By redirecting the parent to a more appropriate and realistic goal, the conversation can be much more productive.

A useful strategy is to role play a parent-child conversation while adhering to rules such as *you need to be supportive but not try to change what I am feeling;* or *try to give comfort not advice.* The idea of comfort is a useful one for parents to have in mind as it relates to helping another person get through a difficulty over which we have no control. A major obstacle for parents in doing this is their own distress at seeing their child in discomfort. The need to help is so strong that the idea of not being able to seems alien. Paradoxically, when parents actually find themselves unable to make practical change in how their child feels, they often become frustrated with the child who is "putting them through this." This frustration is commonly expressed in phrases such as *"You won't let me help you"* or *"You don't want to get better"* or simply *"What do you want from me?"* The child is not supported by these statements. Often, it is after parents relinquish the role of fixer and take up that of comforter that the child begins to experience them as most helpful. To help parents understand this, the therapist can try using the following analogy:

> Imagine that your child came to you and said, "Mommy, I have a really big test this week and I don't feel ready at all." You might respond by saying something like "Well, why don't you study then, and then you'll be ready in time." But imagine that the child seems indifferent to this and instead says: "I really don't feel like studying, I'm just not into it right now and I can't concentrate." You might feel exasperated and say, "Well, I can't study for you. If you don't study that's your choice and you just won't do as well." But then your child looks offended and says, "Don't you care if I do well? I thought you loved me!" At this point all you can think of to say is, "Of course I do, I really think you should study," but right away you're interrupted with, "But I just told you I don't want to study, aren't you even listening to me??"

This snippet of conversation may seem somewhat bizarre but it (and many others like it) actually occurs regularly between parents and children and has its root in what can be termed *confusion of responsibility*. In the slightly exaggerated example above, the child is feeling upset about something and assumes it is the parent's job to alleviate that. The parent has fallen into the trap and has not recognized that they have been charged with an impossible task. There is no "perfect thing to say" that will make the child switch to "Thank you, mom, that was really helpful. You really know how to give great advice!" In fact, parent and child are both aware of the limited options but none of them appeals to the child. A more helpful thing for the parent to say might be, *"It sounds like you really are in a bind. You don't want to study and you want to do well. I wish I could help you with that but I really don't think I can. I hope you think of something."* By reframing the problem as one the child is contending with and not attempting to take responsibility for it, the situation can become defused. Additionally, the child may actually ask for specific help (such as tutoring) that the parent can choose to provide.

REFERENCES

Anderson, E. R., & Hope, D. A. (2008). A review of the tripartite model for understanding the link between anxiety and depression in youth. *Clinical Psychology Review, 28*(2), 275–287.

Beck, A. T., Emery, G., & Greenberg, R. L. (2005). *Anxiety disorders and phobias: A cognitive perspective* (15th anniversary ed.). Cambridge, MA: Basic Books.

Bowlby, J. (1969). *Attachment and loss*. New York, NY: Basic Books.

Dobson, K. S. (1985). The relationship between anxiety and depression. *Clinical Psychology Review, 5*(4), 307–324. doi:10.1016/0272-7358(85) 90010-8

Hewitt, P. L., Caelian, C. F., Flett, G. L., Sherry, S. B., Collins, L., & Flynn, C. A. (2002). Perfectionism in children: Associations with depression, anxiety, and anger. *Personality and Individual Differences, 32* (6), 1049–1061. doi:10.1016/s0191-8869(01)00109-x

Kashdan, T. B. (2007). Social anxiety spectrum and diminished positive experiences: Theoretical synthesis and meta-analysis. *Clinical Psychology Review, 27*(3), 348–365. doi:10.1016/j.cpr.2006.12.003

Kirkcaldy, B. D., Eysenck, M., Furnham, A. F., & Siefen, G. (1998). Gender, anxiety and self-image. *Personality and Individual Differences*, *24*(5), 677–684.

Rowling, J. K. (1999). *Harry Potter and the prisoner of Azkaban*. New York, NY: Levine Books.

PART THREE

Working with Parents

CHAPTER EIGHT

Parental Support and Protection

Support and protection are two important parental functions. Knowing the difference, when to provide which, and how to do so is a major stumbling block for parents of anxious children. This chapter explores the differences between the two roles and presents useful ways of encouraging supportive parenting when overprotection has become the rule.

Key points in this chapter:

- Attachment, separation, and anxiety
- Protection and support
- Protective parenting
- Demanding parenting

ATTACHMENT, SEPARATION, AND ANXIETY

Jane was a 6-year-old girl who had just entered my office for the first time, accompanied by her mom. Jane was visibly nervous; she clung to her mother's arm as she walked into the room and plaintively asked to sit on her own chair. Her thumb made occasional movements toward her mouth, retreating at mom's pointed looks. "Hi there sweetie," I said in a friendly voice. "You must be Jane."

Jane blushed and shook her head forcefully. Leaning over she whispered into her mother's ear, who in turn told me, "She doesn't want you to talk to her," and added, "I knew it would be like this."

This scene must surely be familiar to most clinicians who work with young children, and for those experiencing it for the first time, the situation might seem quite hopeless. How can therapists hope to establish a relationship or even have a conversation with a shy child who won't look at them, much less answer a direct question? But those of us who have been through this particular scenario once or twice before know a secret that neither Jane nor her mother realize yet at this point. The secret is that if, by any means, we are able to get mom to leave the room for a few minutes, it's more than likely that within a short time Jane could be sitting on the rug playing with some dolls, gossiping about the horrible girl in her class, or even talking about the reasons she came in for her appointment.

It seems quite puzzling: A girl is shy and clings to her mom, but actually seems less shy when her parents are out of the room. Curiously, the rule holds not only for shy kids talking to strangers but for many of the other things children are afraid of. A boy will eat only very specific foods, perhaps even insist his parents buy only one particular brand of corn flakes and never eat anything but those (dry with no milk, of course) but then be visiting a friend's house and munch happily on a tuna sandwich without batting an eye. Or a child who is afraid of the dark and will only go to sleep with every light in the house on, night after night, may suddenly sleep over at a friend's and not have any trouble at all. Parents may be very puzzled by these occurrences and could even draw the conclusion that their child is just faking the fear when around them. After all, "If you can do it there, why won't you do it at home?" seems likes a very reasonable question.

Understanding the paradox, whereby children who are anxious will seek their parents' protection, but in the parents' absence will often be less anxious, provides an important key. It offers an insight that can help children and their parents to overcome many of the problematic behavioral patterns that are typical of anxiety disorders. When children are very young they are generally unable to independently cope with most of the dangers and challenges they face in the world. This is particularly so for very young babies who are incapable of fending off any danger on their own. This is true of most mammalian species, and nature has equipped babies with a system to aid them in surviving these treacherous and precarious early stages of life. We are born "programmed" to respond to threat by seeking the protection of those who not only care about us but are also developed enough, physically and cognitively, to keep us safe. We place ourselves in the care of another because of our own fragility and helplessness. Rather than relying on our own, as yet underdeveloped and insufficient resources, we make use of the resources that our caretakers mobilize on our behalf. Natural parental instincts complete the system by ensuring that those caretakers are powerfully motivated to make great personal sacrifice to keep their baby safe from any harm. Although this is not the only solution to the fragility of the newborn (some species solve the problem by having so many offspring that even though an overwhelming majority will perish, enough survive to ensure the continuity of the species), this has long been the mammalian way—for the young to rely on the resources of parents until their own capabilities have developed enough to allow for independence.

This is the key to the paradox: Children often act less capable in their parents' presence because they are accustomed to using their parents as a proxy for their own undeveloped coping mechanisms. As time goes by and children mature, their own abilities will ripen to the point that they are able to handle more and more of the environment independently. Attachment theory (Bowlby, 1969, 1978), which uses the term *attachment* to describe the parent-caretaker bond we have just described, posits that secure attachment with one's parents will lead to a positive view of the world that encourages exploration and a gradual shift toward self-reliance and autonomy.

Unfortunately, many things can hamper this process of maturation. Factors, both environmental and innate, can lead children to view the world more negatively or themselves as less able to rely on their own coping capabilities. Sometimes, difficulty in the regulation of emotion (as discussed in Chapter 2) will predispose a child to anxiety and sensitivity, sometimes negative life experiences may make a child more wary or less self-reliant, and other times the attachment bond itself may be insufficiently sound to allow for the development of autonomy. When these things happen, children will tend to rely more on their parents' ability to protect them from danger or discomfort and less on their own capacity to defend themselves or overcome anxiety. They might see themselves as considerably less able to deal with the world than they actually are. The habit of relying on mom or dad to help get through the anxiety is so persistent that they are likely to miss out on any number of opportunities to discover that they're actually much stronger than they believe.

A story is told about a young boy who visits the circus with his father. The child is amazed at the sight of the powerful elephant standing docilely in the corner attached to a stake by a small rope from which he could clearly break free at any instant. "How come the elephant doesn't just walk away?" he asks. The father explains that when he is very young and not very strong the trainers tie the elephant to the stake with a similar rope but try as he might he isn't strong enough to break free. After trying for a long time the elephant gives up and accepts his limits. As he grows bigger and stronger the elephant never realizes that his circumstances have changed. He continues to view rope, stake, and himself in exactly the same way and never makes any attempt to break free.

Although this tale might expose the difficult fate of circus animals, it is also a powerful metaphor for human nature. For some children the rope just doesn't seem to get any smaller, as they continue to feel helpless or overwhelmed by things they are actually much better prepared to face. There is, however, one difference. The trainer knows that the elephant has matured and that his weakness is purely an illusion that would crumble if put to the test. For many parents the illusion seems like fact, as they perceive their child the same way he sees himself.

How can children discover that they are actually much more capable than they feel with dealing with the challenges or situations that make them anxious? Often it is only when parental protection is withdrawn a little that children may find themselves drawing on their own inner strength. To encourage this in a helpful manner that will strengthen rather than overwhelm their child, it is important for parents to make the distinction between protection and support. A therapist engaged in parent work with the parents of an anxious or fearful child can often use this distinction as a starting point for launching a successful and collaborative course of treatment.

PROTECTION AND SUPPORT

Ask any group of parents what is your most important job as a parent, and *protecting my child from harm* is likely to be up there with the top responses. What more archetypical image of parenting is there than that of a mother lioness fending off attackers who dare to venture too near her cubs? Or of a father standing between his child and danger, putting himself in harm's way to protect the child he loves. These are images of protection and they are well suited to any situation in which a child faces a real and immediate danger. Protecting our children is a primal instinct and an evolutionary dictum. Both of the authors of this book are parents and we would both do anything in our power to protect our children from harm.

But not every situation represents a true danger to a child. As children (and as adults as well) we fear many things that do not pose any real risk at all. Ghosts, darkness, clowns, sounds, speaking to another person, or being alone in a room are all examples of the many things that children may fear dreadfully—although they pose no risk. When a child fears an object or a situation that is not actually dangerous, protection stops being a worthy cause and becomes a liability of its own.

As a therapist I often ask parents the following question: "If what she's afraid of isn't dangerous—what are you actually protecting her from?" Inevitably we end up with the same answer— *We're protecting her from the fear itself!* By protecting a child from fear, parents are effectively teaching them that *fear is dangerous and should be avoided*—Not so! And not helpful, either.

An alternative to protection is **support**. Like protection, support is a primary parental function and it refers to all the ways in which parents bridge the gaps between their children's current abilities and the tasks they face. When children are only partially ready to take on a new challenge, or are faced with a situation that stresses their capabilities, they need the support of their parents to succeed. Over time most tasks become easier and parents take great pleasure observing their child mastering new skills so that their support is no longer necessary.

> Think of your child's first steps. The shaky balance, the weakness of her muscles, the inevitable fall. At first your child probably needed a lot of support to walk. Perhaps you held out your hands for her to fall into? Or maybe you held her hand as she progressed from crawling to supported walking. Either way, you probably soon witnessed her rapid progress to independent walking. Your support—enabling her to challenge herself while still being there when she needed you to pick her up, kiss her bruise, or stabilize her tottering gait—allowed her to make that progress. Imagine if you had said to yourself "She mustn't fall!" If you never allowed her to fall at all you would have had to pick her up and carry her everywhere. She might never have learned to walk. Imagine her growing up thinking she can't walk.

What Is Support?

Supportive responses of parents toward anxious children are achieved when parents successfully integrate two distinct messages:

1. *Acceptance*—I accept that you are afraid and acknowledge that what you are feeling is real and legitimate. I am not trying to deny your experience or to belittle it.
2. *Confidence*—I have faith in your ability. I know you can cope and believe you are strong enough to face this challenge successfully.

As we discuss more fully in Chapter 13 on increasing collaboration between parents, many couples inadvertently split the integrated message into its individual components. One parent takes full responsibility for *acceptance* (and usually also reassurance) and the other is in charge of *confidence* (and perhaps some more aggressive nudging toward coping). When the message is broken up in this way, children are likely to feel confused about what is expected of them and may perceive the more demanding parent as being less caring or loving. Clinging to the reassuring parent in these situations locks them both into corner where any demands for improved coping are translated into act of abandonment or lack of empathy.

Protection	Support
Suitable to real danger	Suitable for challenges
Does not encourage progress	Enables gradual progress and development
Child continues to feel afraid and weak	Allows the child to feel "brave" and competent
Child continues to view situation as dangerous	Child can come to view situation as safe
Parents continue to see child as weak	Parents develop sense of child's ability

An important element of support that differentiates it from both protective and demanding stances is the commitment to gradual progress and to the appreciation of partial accomplishments. By recognizing that the child is truly anxious, the need for immediate and total success is removed. However, by believing in the child's ability to withstand the anxiety, the need for protection is removed and progress becomes possible. The outcome is that a supportive parental stance encourages and strives for gradual forward motion rather than either great leaps or immobility.

One way to introduce parents to the idea of support, rather than protection, is to invite them to imagine how they would like to see their children in one or two years' time: How would they be different? Although any answers are relevant at first, the therapist can try to focus the conversation on the topic of children's anxiety. Will they be less fearful? Perhaps they can imagine them doing that thing they avoid so adamantly? Will they be freer to hang out with friends? To enjoy the things they are missing out on?

Therapist and parents can then engage in some reverse engineering. What has to happen for that scenario to become reality? The therapist should avoid replacing hope with guilt ("Yes, I know we are doing it all wrong") and instead try to help the parents to identify real steps that could bridge the gap between the current situation and the desired future. What supports will children need to go from where they are now to where they would like them to be? What kinds of things may impede the changes envisioned? How can the parents assist in making the fantasy a reality? Through this exercise, parents can understand that their support can promote change and development, whereas protection ensures that things remain the same, or worse, than the current situation.

> The father of a child with OCD, who avoided any exposure to dirt or germs and refused to do any exercise because he immediately felt the need to shower at length, gave the following description:

> "I see our son running on the baseball field. He has his hand up in the air to catch a ball and his uniform is covered in mud from the great slide he made last play. He's completely focused on catching that ball and I can see he's going to make it."

> The scene represented a fantasy to him because at present his child could never be completely focused on any one thing—He always needed to monitor his environment for any sign of danger. In this case the vigilance was focused on exposure to germs or dirt. Of course, he would never have agreed to wearing anything with dirt or to sliding in the mud.

> In order for that dream to come true, the father realized that his son would have to come to believe that he was able to withstand the "terrible" sensations of being dirty. As long as he felt unable to bear them he would need to continue his avoidance—and goodbye to baseball.

Other elements of support, discussed and operationalized in more detail throughout this section of the book, are the willingness to promote change without requiring the child's insight or agreement. The willingness to create a broader support network that includes more than only the parents or siblings. And the explicit acceptance of the fact that although parents can want the best for their child, they cannot, and will not try, to directly control the child's behavior or feelings.

When children experience parents as supportive rather than protective, they are more likely to change the way they see themselves. When we ask children suffering from anxiety to describe themselves, they rarely will use words like brave, strong, courageous, or competent. Not surprisingly, they are much more likely to choose adjectives like weak, cowardly, or afraid. Inherent in overcoming anxiety is a change in this self-perception. In the absence of support, such a self-perceptual shift is unlikely.

Confidence Alone—The Demanding Parent

Many parents will find it easier to believe in their child's ability to cope than to accept the face that their child is afraid. They will consistently express confidence in the child's ability, but will avoid explicit recognition of the challenges faced by the child. Statements that are typical of demanding parents include:

- If we baby her she'll never get over it.
- How do I get him to do this already?
- I'm not sure that he's not really just trying to get attention.
- We shouldn't give in to this nonsense.

Children who perceive that their parents do not acknowledge their feelings are usually going to be continually preoccupied with proving that they indeed feel what they say. Indeed, if overcoming anxiety is tantamount to admitting to having been "faking it" or being "babyish," they will resist this change as strongly as they can. For this reason, when faced with an overly demanding parent, many children will "dig in with both feet," and rather than moving toward a more positive sense of competence and ability, will become greatly invested in defending their feelings of fear and anxiety. Positive statements such as "You can do this" are experienced as challenges to their integrity or as an attempt to dictate their inner state, and they respond defensively by insisting on their weaknesses, which in turn is seen by adults as unwillingness to overcome their problem. This is one manner in which a nonsupportive message can hamper communication and lessen the chances of increased coping.

Often in this situation, the demanding parent who relies exclusively on *confidence* without integrating acceptance to create a supportive whole, will become frustrated and feel inclined to disengage from the issue entirely. The message turns from "You can do this" into "Do this— or I give up," and the child feels helpless and alone. Although stemming from positive sentiments and intentions, demanding parenting is usually not able to help children view themselves more positively. In fact, in addition to insisting outwardly on the veracity of their emotions, inwardly children may actually feel even weaker than before. The message of demand implies that not being able to fulfill those expectations is a sign of great weakness and the child experiences failure, reinforcing the self-image of helplessness and inadequacy.

Below are some questions that can serve to identify the demanding pattern in parents and launch the discussion about the issue:

- Do you tell your child that all his fears are groundless, and he should stop it with the nonsense?
- Do you reprimand her for her anxious reactions?
- Do you think, or say, that her anxiety is a show or a manipulation?
- Do you believe the whole problem can be solved by just presenting him with a firm and decisive demand?
- Do you sometimes give up and prefer to just avoid the issue?

Working with an Overly Demanding Parent

For many clinicians, the demanding parent presents unique dilemmas and challenges. As behavioral therapists, who recognize the importance of exposure and want to foster coping rather than avoidance, a parent who emphasizes confidence may seem like the perfect ally—and will often eventually be a vital collaborator in the therapeutic process, but only after successfully integrating acceptance to form a more supportive stance. Additionally, the therapist needs to avoid presenting a confusing message that would appear to negate the idea of the child's inner strength.

A related obstacle is discussed more fully in Chapter 13 on fostering collaboration between parents. For many couples, one parent's insistence on coping and meeting challenges is a thorny issue that has already been the source of much contention in the couple's relationship. Therapists need to be wary of becoming identified with one side of an ongoing disagreement, particularly as both sides of this particular quarrel probably represent positive and important elements of supporting the child. By allowing themselves to be seen as bolstering the sentiments of one parent, therapists can easily forfeit the trust of the other. When this happens, the therapeutic sessions can quickly provide fuel for more disagreement.

Many of the more demanding parents we have worked with have also tended to be among those more wary of placing their trust in the practitioners and maxims of modern psychology. The need to gain or retain the trust of parents is ever a factor in the clinical work of treating children. Parents who are by nature more stoically oriented often enter into the process of parent counseling with a caution and vigilance for "psychological pampering."

Bearing these challenges in mind, therapists should attempt to emphasize their acknowledgment of the value inherent in the demanding parent's views as well as their recognition of the positive wishes that underlie them. As is helpful in many other contexts, however, it may be necessary to challenge the efficacy of attempting to act as they have done in the past. Questions such as, "So how's that working out for you?," when asked with a smile, can help to raise the issue of the discrepancy between the positive goals and the efficacy of the means.

For some overly demanding parents, it is useful to consider areas or times in their life in which they have experienced anxiety themselves. Thinking back to what was useful to them and to how they felt about different kinds of reactions they encountered or advice they received can be a good way to steer the conversation toward more useful kinds of responses. Some parents will resist the idea that they have contended with anxiety or "surrendered to it." One father, who was a war veteran, when asked to think back to the fear the members of his squadron surely experienced under attack stated decisively: *"Some were afraid — but I slapped them on their helmets and told them not to be wimps!"* A potentially useful strategy on the battlefield, but not particularly useful for his 7-year-old son. Most parents, however, can readily identify anxiety as a component in their lives, and bringing to mind the character of a person whom they trusted and who was helpful to them is a useful way of discussing the necessary elements of support.

Acceptance Alone — The Protective Parent

Parents who accept their children's fears and recognize their validity but are unable to couple that acceptance with a belief in the child's ability to cope with the anxiety or with anxiety-provoking situations are likely to adopt a protective stance toward the child. Any mom or dad who sees their children as weak, helpless, or in danger will be driven inexorably to protect them from danger. This kind of protection, while also stemming from love for the child and positive motivation, is not supportive because it does not offer the child a path toward greater ability and self-confidence.

The irony of protective parenting is that a parent can spend endless energy, time, and resources on reassuring the child without ever making any headway on actually helping the child to become less anxious. In fact, the protective responses may actually be serving to make the anxiety disorder tragically worse. As discussed earlier, a core element in any anxiety disorder is the belief on the part of the child that they are unable to cope with the anxious feelings and reactions and must avoid them at all costs. Parents who react protectively, with the best of intentions, may be reinforcing this belief on the part of their child.

Some typical statements made by protective parents include:

- He's just not strong enough to deal with it.
- I don't want her to be scarred by anxiety.
- I know it's wrong, but I just can't handle seeing her that way.
- I'm afraid of what will happen if we push too hard.

One of the most important adaptations that babies and children bring with them into the world is an innate tendency to learn what is safe and what is dangerous. Without this predisposition all children would have to "learn through their own mistakes" about the dangers of everything from snakes to fire to electrical outlets. Luckily, nature has endowed us with the ability to observe the reactions of our parents and save a lot of trials and errors in experimenting with the environment. An implication of this important system, however, is that as children we are very vulnerable to adopting unrealistic fears held by our parents. If a parent reacts with visible anxiety to a given situation, children are likely to quickly learn that the situation is best avoided.

A protective parent, who displays a powerful emotional reaction to a child who is experiencing fear, can send a very powerful message. The message is: "What you feel right now is actually very dangerous—you should never ever let yourself feel that way again." Unfortunately, it is entirely unrealistic to eliminate fear from a child's life, and the outcome can be a parent and child who together collaborate to avoid all possible experiences of anxiety—and end up constantly afraid.

Below are some questions that can serve to identify the protective pattern in parents and launch the discussion about them:

- Do you feel like it's your job to protect your child from anxiety?
- Do you believe feeling anxious is harmful to your child?
- Do you feel like only you really get what your child is going through?
- Do you try to help your child to avoid situations that will cause her to feel afraid?
- Do you think your child will grow out of his fears if he is not forced to confront them before he's ready?

Working with an Overly Protective Parent

No parent will be able to benefit from counseling unless trust is established between parent and therapist. Such trust can be difficult to establish when a parent's role as their child's protector is being challenged. It is important that the parents understand that the therapist identifies with their need to ensure the child's well-being and is fully committed to that goal. Establishing this can be key to overcoming the parents' misgivings. It may be useful to explicitly state the recognition of the parent's protective role and goal. An example of such a statement could be:

> I understand that you would do anything to protect your child and I admire that. You are willing to make tremendous personal sacrifice to keep your child safe from harm and there is no more worthy goal for a parent in my eyes. I want you to understand that I share that goal as well. I will not make any recommendations to you that I think could cause any damage. Although some things we do may make your child uncomfortable, they will not hurt him.

Children suffering from anxiety often fear that the treatment will progress too fast or they will be expected to take big steps or to progress more rapidly than they feel able. Parents can share the same kinds of apprehension. Helping a parent to understand that the treatment can progress very gradually and no one is being "thrown into the river to learn to swim" can also lower resistance and alleviate apprehension.

An important part of shifting away from a protective role and toward a more supportive one lies in recognition of the need for change. Using the kind of "backward engineering" we described earlier, or otherwise stimulating a conversation about the problems with the current approach, will be a necessary step in the treatment process.

For some parents, adopting a protective stance will stem from their own experience of anxiety or fear, whether in the past or the present. Many adults grew up feeling anxious, afraid, worried, or shy without receiving the recognition or acceptance that is a vital part of any supportive approach. For these parents, acceptance may seem like the only element that was missing and they may be determined not to allow their own child to suffer from the same lonely experience. Tina, speaking about her experience of social anxiety disorder as a child, told me:

> I waited, day after day, for someone to notice that I was unhappy. I asked myself how they can be so blind. I remember playing with my dolls and my favorite game was to line them all up and ask each one how they felt. Who had a stomachache, who hurt themselves, and who was unhappy? I heard grown-ups describe me as a shy girl and I wanted to yell at them "Calling me shy doesn't make it any better," but I never had the voice to say it. I swore to myself that when I was a mother I would know everything my child was feeling. That not a day would go by that I wouldn't ask my kid if there was anything wrong and that if there was, I would fix it.

After Tina shared her experiences with me, I was able to better understand why she felt so compelled to protect her son from feeling anxious, and why she responded so protectively when he was upset or afraid. We went on, though, to discuss that the idea that although acceptance might have been the thing she missed the most as a child, what that little girl really needed was not just someone to ask her what was wrong or to recognize that she was in pain. She also needed someone, a grown-up with maturity and experience, to tell her how to make it better. She had become so fixated on ensuring that her son didn't feel alone that she forgot he needed more than comforting. He needed to know how to get better.

Many parents are acutely aware that protection alone is not enough. In our work we frequently encounter parents who say: "I know it's wrong for me to react like this, but I'm just not able to behave differently when I see him so upset." Parents who make this kind of statement are probably feeling guilty and defeated and are often subjecting themselves to a lot of self-criticism. They may also be the targets of criticism from others, such as a frustrated spouse. Adding one more voice to the chorus of accusatory notes is unlikely to be of any real help to them. A little like the frazzled mom whose child is throwing a temper tantrum in a supermarket because she wants that candy bar, parents can be aware that "giving in" is not helpful while feeling unable to act differently. Parents who feel this way need empathy and support no less than their child who is struggling with anxiety. Just like support for a child is only possible when it integrates the need for change and the belief in its feasibility with an acceptance of the conditions and emotions that are currently dominant, support for a parent also requires both elements. Accusations of inefficacy, even when worded politely or euphemistically, are more likely to cause a parent to react defensively (*"That's easy for you to say—you don't know what it's like"*) than to elicit the inner strength necessary for changing behavioral patterns.

REFERENCES

Bowlby, J. (1969). *Attachment and loss*. New York, NY: Basic Books.
Bowlby, J. (1978). Attachment theory and its therapeutic implications. *Adolescent Psychiatry, 6*, 5–33.

CHAPTER NINE

Childhood Anxiety and Family Boundaries

The boundaries between parents and anxious children tend to become blurred, leading to enmeshment that can make coping more difficult. This chapter explores different aspects of family boundaries and the ways that supportive parents can reestablish healthy separation.

Key points in this chapter:

- How anxiety can affect the personal boundary.
- Four aspects of the parents' boundaries.
- The protective parent and family boundaries.
- The demanding and family boundaries.

THE PERSONAL BOUNDARY

The gradual separation and individualization of children from their parents is such a core part of human development that it has been the focus of theoreticians (not to mention parents) again and again (Bowlby, 1978; Edward, Ruskin, & Turrini, 1992; Kaplan, 1978; Mahler, 1968). We all come into this world highly dependent on our parents, and even relatively short periods of separation can be mortally dangerous to us in these early stages of life. Indeed, prior to birth comes a period of even greater dependence as a fetus grown inside its mother is completely dependent and at one with her.

But all too quickly, the process of separation begins and picks up speed as child and parents live their deeply linked yet separate lives, and parents gradually become less totally accessible to their offspring. For some, this process is relatively easy as both parents and child take naturally to the separation and thrive in their individual domains of existence. For others, the process may be painful and challenging, fraught with anxiety or the need to resist any evidence of mounting distance. Parent and child alike may find separation to be a source of distress and prefer to delay its advance when possible. But for most families, as children grow and their immediate needs diminish, parents will become less completely accessible.

The personal boundary can be thought of as an imaginary line created by and representative of all the ways in which parents express to their children the fact that that they are indeed separate individuals, with limited accessibility. Behaviors, spoken messages, rules, even beliefs and expectations, all contribute to the parents' personal boundaries and convey to the child that they love the child and are willing to do anything for them—but they are not a part of them.

ANXIETY AND FAMILY BOUNDARIES

When a child is naturally fearful or is suffering from an anxiety disorder, establishing and maintaining a healthy personal boundary can be particularly challenging. Helping parents to reestablish boundaries, to set healthy limits on their own accessibility to the child, can be a major stumbling block to the advance of treatment. As we discussed in the previous chapter, anxious children who see themselves as less able to take on the responsibilities of coping with the world will often rely more heavily on their parents for this purpose, leading to gradual erosion of the personal boundaries. The concept of parents as safe harbor to which to return, as described in attachment theory (Bowlby, 1969), is dependent on the capacity for at least temporary separation. It requires the establishment of boundaries between parent and child. Other theoretical perspectives have used other languages to describe the varied ways in which a child's anxiety can cause or be caused by difficulty in creating and maintaining healthy boundaries appropriate to the child's age (Kerr & Bowen, 1988; P. Minuchin, 1985; S. Minuchin, 1982; Olson, 2011; Wood, 1985).

It is important to remember that a healthy personal boundary does not mean total separation or complete inaccessibility of the parents to a child. Parents will and should continue to remain accessible even to grown children. Different kinds of stress and various needs will trigger greater closeness and dependence in a fluid and dynamic pattern. Parents and children are truly connected in a multitude of ways, and it is for this reason that personal boundaries are so important. Just as maintaining clear borders is only an issue between contiguous and related geographical entities, parents and children need clear personal boundaries exactly because they are never detached or disconnected.

To assess the degree to which a parent's personal boundaries have become vague or indistinct, here are some questions that probe the various aspects of the personal boundary:

- Is your time your own or has it been taken over by your child's anxiety? For example, is your work schedule compromised by the need to be with your child because of her fears? Are you spending much time on reassuring her because she is anxious?
- Has your personal space shrunk because of your child's anxiety? For example, does your child insist on sleeping in your bed? Does he need unlimited access to you physically or by phone? Does he object to your closing the door?
- Do you feel anxious when your child feels anxious? Do you feel overwhelmed or like you need to do something right away to make it better?
- Are you doing more and more things for your child instead of his doing them himself? Is your day-to-day life dictated by your child's anxiety or by his limitations?
- Are you able to keep your child from interrupting you during conversations or other activities because of her anxiety?
- Do you feel entitled to your own plans and wishes? Are you able to realize those plans?

141

Dimensions of the Personal Boundary

Personal boundaries between parents and children have many manifestations. These include physical separation in space, their independent management of time, and their distinct behaviors and emotions.

Space

Perhaps the most basic aspect of any boundary is that of spatial separation, and parental boundaries are no exception. In the famous psychological experiments conducted by Harry Harlow (Harlow & Zimmermann, 1959) to study what he termed the *affectional patterns* of young monkeys, fear was used to elicit the predictable attachment response—physical clinging to the mother figure. Young mammals, including humans, who are afraid tend to cling to their caretakers. And anxious children will often shadow their parents so closely that boundaries seem like a long ago memory. Even children whose primary diagnosis is not one of separation anxiety disorder are likely to prefer to spend as much time as possible very near their parents, for the reassurance and comfort they provide. Closed doors, physical manifestations of separateness and space, are often abhorred by anxious children. They might feel compelled to shower or use the toilet with the door open because of the fear they experience, or they may react with acute fear to the closed door to a parent's room.

Parents who lose their personal space because of the child's fear may harbor some resentment toward the child because of the deprivation of privacy or sleep, but they might hesitate to express this for fear of sounding uncaring or harsh. As discussed in the previous chapter, an understanding of the parent's role as supporter rather than protector of the child can help to frame the parents' needs as being in line with those of the child rather than in conflict with them.

Time

The way we spend our time is a basic aspect of who we are, and from the moment we become parents our time is rarely truly our own. Phone calls from school, a child with a fever, or just watching a kid's program on TV are all ways in which parents may find some of their time "taken over" by their parenthood—and this is completely normal. However, a child's anxiety has a way of eating away ever larger chunks of time often, leaving parents with the feeling of having no personal time at all. When parents' personal boundaries are eroded because of children's anxiety, they may find that their time has been gradually taken over by the need to reassure the child or to prevent situations in which they are likely to feel anxiety. They may spend hours doing things that would normally be the child's responsibility, or staying home with a child who is afraid to stay alone.

Joanne was a good worker who had held the same job in a small local bank for many years. She dreamed of holding a higher position that would bring with it more financial freedom and greater responsibility, but in fact she had been passed over for promotion numerous times. Joanne was obviously a bright and energetic woman with good social skills, so her lack of promotion seemed surprising. She explained:

"It's no mystery. Every time my name comes up for promotion it's the same thing. I have a talk with my supervisor and things go well until I start thinking about Don. Don is 16 now but is still unable to spend any time by himself. A few years ago he suffered from panic attacks and since that time he has been terrified of having an attack when no one is home. He hasn't had an attack in years, but he's just so afraid. Until this year he needed me to meet him at the bus stop outside our house and walk in with him. Now he's made some progress and walks in by himself, but if I'm not there to greet him he'll freak out. A promotion always means some trips here and there or working late some afternoons and I just can't do that to him. Not when he's finally made some progress."

Joanne's concern for her son was understandable and her willingness to make personal sacrifice on his behalf was laudable, but her choices reflected a personal boundary that had become overly permeable. Her time was controlled by the need to allow her son to continue acting in an avoidant way, which ironically greatly diminished the chances of his overcoming his anxiety disorder. Joanne feared that if she made a decision to use her time in a way that reflected her own needs rather than his, she would bring about a regression in Don's condition or a recurrence of his panic attacks. In fact, although a panic attack may have occurred, it is far more likely that he would have discovered himself to be much better able to handle her absence than either of them believed.

Actions

Nothing can reflect our individuality more than what we do, and losing a sense of personal agency, feeling like one's behavior is controlled by another, is a difficult and distressing experience. Parents of anxious children have often described to us the sensation of being "more an extension of their child than their own person" or acting like "a third arm of the child" used to achieve an escape from anxiety and fear. We explored this issue in greater detail in Chapter 3 on family accommodation.

Actions that parents perform because of their child's anxiety may include:

Doing things the child is afraid to do on his or her own, such as speaking to a shopkeeper, getting something from the basement, touching a doorknob (for a child who is afraid of germs).

Doing things with the child because he or she is afraid to do them on his or her own, such as staying at a party because the child won't stay alone, or sleeping in the child's bed.

Doing things the child needs done to feel reassured, such as checking the lock on doors, or repeating good night rituals.

Some of the most dramatic examples of parents' behavior being dictated by children's anxiety occur in the context of a child's obsessive-compulsive disorder. Children suffering from OCD will perform many rituals aimed at reducing their anxiety and dispelling feelings of distress. For many children it is natural to involve their parents in their rituals and parents will often begin to feel as if they are the ones with the OCD rather than the child.

Tim, a young father to 7-year-old Jacob, told me about how he became part of the OCD rituals:

When Jacob starting worrying about germs he developed a lot of rules about when he would need to wash his hands and just how many times he needed to wash each one before he felt sure they were clean. Eating in particular was a huge problem. Whenever he needed to eat anything he would get stuck in these washing rituals and sometimes would have to stop eating in the middle and start them all over again for fear of eating something contaminated with germs.

One evening I was preparing his dinner, macaroni and cheese, and he was sitting there watching me. He was upset because he knew as soon as dinner was ready he'd have to start on his washing and he was feeling tired of it. All of a sudden he said to me "Dad, I could wash really well but it won't help if the food is dirty. Did you wash your hands before you started cooking?" from that moment he was relentless. He would ask me again and again if I'd washed my hands. If I refused to answer he got so upset and wouldn't eat anything at all. He'd say I don't love him or don't care about him. Eventually I started lying about how many times I washed and eventually he caught me. Now he insists I wash my hands in front of him just like he does or he won't eat anything at all. My hands are red and raw from all the washing but I just don't know how to stop without hurting him.

Feelings
Sometimes, the boundaries between parents and children suffering from anxiety become frayed, not only in the more practical and pragmatic aspects like time space and action, but in much more delicate and subtle ways such as the emotional boundaries that separate what one person is feeling from another's emotional experience. When parents' emotional boundaries have become permeable they may feel swept away by the child's feelings, or as if the fear has become contagious and has infected them as well.

Empathy, being able to place yourself in "someone else's shoes" and develop a sense for what they might be experiencing, is a core aspect of human interpersonal relationships and all the more so in the intimate relationship between parent and child. But empathy is not about experiencing the same thing as the other person. Empathic parents will be able to understand what their child is feeling but can still maintain a boundary that denotes it as *the child's* experience, rather than their own. A useful metaphor to explain this point to parents focuses on the loss of the ability to help a child, when parent and child share the same experience:

> Imagine you are out hiking with your child in a field outside your home. You're walking alone, the sun will soon be setting, and your child stumbles into a deep pit in the ground. There is no way for him to climb out alone, so without thinking you jump right in and sit down next to him. Now your child is no longer alone. Unfortunately you are now both stuck in the pit without any way of getting out or calling for help. The hardest thing in the world would have been to say to your child "I know how afraid you must feel but I am going to get help so we can get out of here and go back home together." But that was also the best way to help the two of you get out of the trap they've fallen into.

For many parents the ability to say to a child "I understand what you are feeling—but I am feeling something different" is the hardest thing of all. It may feel like abandonment rather than support, but it is helpful to remind parents that it is also the best way to give the child help. A permeable boundary allows the anxiety to flow both ways. Just as parents may feel overwhelmed by their child's anxiety the anxious emotion, reflected back to the child in the parent's eyes, can only serve to increase the fear they were already experiencing. For many children there is nothing more frightening than being gripped by fear and seeing your parents looking just as panicked!

> Anita was a 9-year-old girl who suffered from panic disorder and would experience sudden acute episodes of terror during which she was convinced she was dying. Each attack looked alike. Anita would start to feel shortness of breath and could tell that her pulse was quickening. Her body would become covered in a sheen of sweat and her skin would rapidly change color, going pale and then flushed in rapid succession. Anita's parents were terrified of her attacks. Her mother, Shana, had been with her to the hospital emergency room on a number of occasions and had heard the same thing every time. Her daughter was physically healthy and was suffering from an anxiety disorder. There was no risk to her health from the attacks themselves. Do not bring her to the hospital next time.

Shana told me she had tried to follow the doctor's instructions but she found that she could not. Not taking her to be checked felt like too big a risk. What if the doctors were wrong? She felt completely overwhelmed by the panic. In addition, she said she did not feel she could do that to her daughter. "I can't not take her," she explained. "How would you feel if you told your parents you were dying and they did nothing? Even if there is no real risk, even if it really is all in her head—I can't have her feel like I don't care."

During our next session Anita came with her mother to the appointment. I asked her to describe to her mother what it felt like to be rushed to the hospital when she has an attack. "It tells me that I really am dying," she said quietly to her mother. "When we go running out the door to the car, I look at you and I think: This is it . . . if my mother who is always in control is so frightened I must really be dying. I know the doctors are wrong because otherwise you wouldn't be so scared."

The Personal Boundary and Protective Parenting

Protective parents create boundaries that are overly permeable and undefined between themselves and their anxious child. As the child becomes increasingly avoidant and dependent on the parent for reassurance, limitations on the parent's accessibility fade. For some protective parents, the very idea of boundaries separating them from their child, particularly during times of heightened anxiety, may seem irrelevant or even repugnant. But as we have discussed, in the absence of such boundaries the child's ability to muster the necessary strength to develop autonomous coping skills is greatly diminished.

One outcome of the overly permeable boundaries between protective parents and anxious children is that other influences, including many potentially positive ones, are "locked out" of the equation. As the parent takes on the role of constant protector, any voice that contradicts the need for such protection or calls for firmer boundaries can be excluded. This is true for a spouse, relative, or friend who is ignored—but it can also be true for a therapist who attempts to change the dynamic. Only with considerable support and trust will such a voice be heard or acted on.

One related challenge is that after prolonged protection, during which parent and child felt that those calling for the child to cope more independently were misunderstanding their reality, it is easy for the parent to feel guilty over "joining forces" with them. Children will often express this sentiment very clearly, accusing the parent of betrayal or abandonment. It is necessary to explore these feelings and prepare supportive statements the parent can make to the child, to express their understanding of how difficult a process is underway, as well as their commitment to doing it for the child's good.

The Personal Boundary and Demanding Parenting

Demanding parents, too, have difficulty maintaining healthy and appropriate boundaries between themselves and their anxious children. For the demanding parent, the boundary can be skewed in two ways. In one case the boundaries of the demanding parent can be overly rigid and impermeable. Although accessibility should be reasonable and limited, children really do need their parents' reassurance, understanding, and closeness. Parents who are frustrated because a child "refuses to buck up" or is being "a sissy" may react with detachment and a lack of involvement that is just as unhealthy as an overly enmeshed and protective boundary. A father who was feeling frustrated with the lack of progress in his son's treatment once said to me, "I give him one more week to stop being afraid—after that he's on his own!" As parents walk away from a situation that is making them feel angry or ineffective, the child is left alone in isolation.

Another kind of reaction typical of overly demanding parents is an attempt to define for the child what their inner experience should be. Typical statements that reflect this stance include:

- Don't be afraid.
- You don't really feel like that.
- That's not frightening.
- You could do this—if you wanted to.

All of these statements represent an attempt on the part of parents to tell the children what they feel, or what they should be feeling. Unfortunately, few people take well to attempts to dictate their inner emotions. Such an attempt represents another kind of breakdown of the personal boundary. We have seen how, when a boundary is unclear, parent and child can transfer emotions to each other in potentially negative ways. In a similar fashion, telling a child what to feel is a denial of the fact that the child is a separate person with his or her own inner feelings. It is as if the parent is saying, "I cannot accept you having feelings that are so different from mine—so now you have to change yours." A more supportive statement would be, "I recognize that you have your own feelings—but I am sure you can overcome them and come to feel less afraid than you do now."

REFERENCES

Bowlby, J. (1969). *Attachment and loss*. New York, NY: Basic Books.

Bowlby, J. (1978). Attachment theory and its therapeutic implications. *Adolescent Psychiatry, 6*, 5–33.

Edward, J., Ruskin, N., & Turrini, P. (1992). *Separation/individuation: Theory and application* (2nd ed.). New York, NY: Brunner/Mazel.

Harlow, H. F., & Zimmermann, R. R. (1959). Affectional responses in the infant monkey; orphaned baby monkeys develop a strong and persistent attachment to inanimate surrogate mothers. *Science, 130*(3373), 421–432.

Kaplan, L. J. (1978). *Oneness and separateness: From infant to individual*. New York, NY: Simon & Schuster.

Kerr, M. E., & Bowen, M. (1988). *Family evaluation: An approach based on Bowen theory* (1st ed.). New York, NY: Norton.

Mahler, M. S. (1968). *On human symbiosis and the vicissitudes of individuation*. New York, NY: International Universities Press.

Minuchin, P. (1985). Families and individual development: Provocations from the field of family therapy. *Child Development, 56*(2), 289–302.

Minuchin, S. (1982). Reflections on boundaries. *American Journal of Orthopsychiatry, 52*(4), 655–663.

Olson, D. (2011). FACES IV and the Circumplex model: Validation study. *Journal of Marital and Family Therapy, 37*(1), 64–80. doi:10.1111/j.1752–0606.2009.00175.x

Wood, B. (1985). Proximity and hierarchy: Orthogonal dimensions of family interconnectedness. *Family Process, 24*(4), 487–507.

CHAPTER TEN

Introduction to Parent Work and the SPACE Program

Many children are too anxious to willingly engage in the kind of treatment described in the preceding chapters. The prospect of overcoming anxiety seems too far out of reach and the idea of facing exposure situations is simply too frightening to undertake. Parents can assume a leadership role—initiating a process of overcoming anxiety rather than waiting helplessly for their child's motivation to surge. In the following chapters we describe a step-by-step treatment protocol for working with parents of anxious children, even (though not exclusively) when the child is not a willing participant in the process.

While he was working in a large anxiety clinic at a busy children's hospital some years ago, Eli Lebowitz, one of the authors, had the job of telephonically screening new cases to assess their suitability for treatment. There were simply too many calls to see everyone, and it was necessary to try to assess who was likely to actually end up being treated in the clinic. Various factors enabled us to guess at who would be a likely candidate. Parents who stated there was no way they could make regular appointments, for example, were probably not potential patients. One important question we always asked was, "Does your child want help?" This was basic because we knew that a child who did not want to get better was unlikely to do well in behavioral treatment. We would explain to the disappointed parents that perhaps in the future their child would feel differently, but at this point, behavioral therapy was probably not going to be helpful. Unfortunately, this left a great many parents asking "Well then, what should I be doing?"

WHY SOME CHILDREN DON'T COOPERATE WITH TREATMENT

There are quite a few reasons for children not to want to collaborate with cognitive behavioral therapy for an anxiety disorder—even when that disorder is significant or causing them a great deal of distress. Some of these reasons include:

Fear that treatment won't help. Some children voice this fear explicitly and a great many others probably experience it inwardly. Without a sense of hope that their efforts will pay off, children are naturally resistant towards an undertaking that will require much work and seems likely to end in failure. An outcome of parent work in these cases can be to provide the child with the experience of improvement or mastery, which can increase their confidence and motivation to collaborate with treatment.

Fear of what treatment will entail. Understanding of the principles of behavioral therapy, including the idea of exposure, is important to the treatment process—but for some children it will also be enough to determine that they are dead set against it! Most anxious children have been completely focused on avoiding those very stimuli, and confronting them can seem too daunting an undertaking. Some children might feel that even if taking initial small steps toward exposure could be possible, these will quickly lead to other much more frightening demands, which they are not willing to face. Through their work, parents can demonstrate their commitment to gradual progress at a pace that will not overwhelm the child.

Depression and other related disorders. Unsurprisingly, many children suffering from anxiety disorders also present with comorbid mood disorders such as depression. Although the causes for this kind of comorbidity are not sufficiently well established, and may vary from case to case, it is likely that the prolonged behavioral inhibition and ongoing stress of chronic anxiety can lead to depression. In turn, depression can bring about a sense of hopelessness and a lack of motivation that can impede participation in treatment. In such cases, postponing any intervention until the child is willing to get to work can result in a protracted course of illness.

Family accommodation. For some children, the cause of resistance to treatment is the sense of having a better, easier way of not feeling anxious. This will usually be a system of avoidance that allows the child to avoid any situation that would otherwise provoke the anxiety. Parental accommodation is almost always a factor in enabling such systematic avoidance. Children suffering from separation anxiety, for instance, will be much less motivated to work on the issue if their parents never leave them alone, than if they are forced to endure uncomfortable separations. Even serious implications for the child's ability to engage in pleasant or desirable activities will often not be enough to motivate treatment when consistent avoidance is a viable option enabled by the child's environment. Clearly, in this case, working with the parents to curtail accommodation may be a necessary precondition to effective work with the child.

Parent-child relationships. From doing their homework to brushing their teeth to cleaning their rooms, children have lots of practice resisting suggestions they perceive as parental impositions on their freedom. Sometimes parent-child relationships are so embattled that even a child who is suffering will prefer to say no than to acquiesce to something that is perceived as a parent's interest. In some cases, the therapist takes on the role of one more grown-up in their lives who, along with parents, teachers, and coaches, is trying to get them to do another kind of chore. Given the nature of behavioral treatment and its emphasis on practicing skills and doing homework, this kind of perception can be destructive to the therapeutic process. By starting parent work without waiting for the child's collaboration, parents convey the message, "Even if you can't work with us yet, we won't give up on you. You are so important to us that we will do our duty and help you by stopping to give in to the anxiety." This can change the conditions that perpetuate the anxiety and possibly increase the chances for future collaboration.

Feeling like they've already tried. Having previously attempted therapy, whether cognitive behavioral or otherwise oriented, and having been disappointed can play a big role in discouraging a child from starting a new therapeutic process. Although there may be good reasons why one therapist might succeed where another has not, the child may feel like they've already "done that"—and to no avail. In this situation, parents' work can be particularly helpful. By coaching parents to take steps that are actually quite different from those that are familiar from the past, a child's curiosity may be piqued and new interest sparked along with the hope that this time things may be different.

Fear of stigmatization. Many children will resist treatment because of a fear of stigmatization or due to negative associations they have to the idea of being in treatment. Despite tremendous progress in this field over the past years, many children (and sadly quite a few adults as well) still hold negative or prejudicial attitudes toward therapy. Only a few years ago it was practically unheard of (in our experience) for a child to independently ask for psychotherapy. Today this happens on a regular basis, as children learn from popular media and other sources that psychologists can help children overcome many problems. However, some children and adolescents still associate treatment with weakness, mental illness (*"I'm not crazy"*), or a frightening and intrusive process. Others are internally prepared to be in therapy but fear real or imagined social repercussions should others discover they needed it.

The SPACE Program

The SPACE Program is a treatment protocol developed at the Yale University Child Study Center and Tel Aviv University, to help parents better support their anxious child and to treat childhood anxiety without direct participation of the child in therapy. The word SPACE in the name of the program is an abbreviation of Supportive Parenting for Anxious Childhood Emotions. The concept of support has been described and discussed in detail in the preceding chapters and the program offers a practical and concrete way of helping parents to translate that principle into action.

The guiding principles of the program are recognition of the authenticity of the anxiety experienced by both child and parents, and a belief in the ability of both to overcome this anxiety, leading to improved coping for the child and increased well-being for the entire family. Parents who participate in the SPACE Program undergo an enormous and meaningful change in their attitudes toward their child and toward themselves as parents. For the children, parents come to see that they are significantly stronger, more capable, and more competent individuals. For themselves, parents learn that they have not only the responsibility but also the capacity to act on behalf of their child. In a study conducted at the Yale Child Study Center, including the parents of children with various anxiety disorders, parents reported significantly less anxiety symptoms in their children following participation in the SPACE Program. In fact, although the treatment focuses on reducing the children's symptoms, parents also reported that their own anxiety was reduced after treatment.

Parents of children suffering from anxiety who are reluctant to participate in treatment such as cognitive behavior therapy or medication, or who have tried these approaches unsuccessfully, often feel an unbearable sense of helplessness, frustration, and exasperation. For parents, seeing their children's limited functioning and emotional distress, without the ability to help them to get better, is a dreadful predicament. The SPACE Program aims to create a shift in the parents' perception of the problem—allowing them to regain the sense of self-efficacy that has been forfeited. Over the course of the SPACE Program parents not only take positive action to increase their children's ability to cope with anxiety and self-regulate their inner state, they also are helped to repair some of the harm that the prolonged anxiety may have caused to their relationship with the children. As parents move from a stance of helplessness toward one of active leadership, they often find that their child seems almost to have been waiting for them to make that change. Parents, who are often convinced their child will resent their unilateral commitment to change and the actions they take in the course of the SPACE Program, may be amazed at the sense of relief the child exhibits. The next two chapters describe the course of the SPACE Program in detail and can be used as a manual by therapists for implementing it with parents.

CHAPTER ELEVEN

The SPACE Program— Treatment Process

Overview and Use of This Manual

The SPACE Program (*Supportive Parenting for Anxious Childhood Emotions*) manual is designed to allow the clinician a blend of structure and flexibility. The treatment follows a structured path, leading to decreased family accommodation of a child's anxiety and better parental support, while allowing the therapist to implement particular tools and strategies based on the characteristics of each case. No two children are alike and the therapist must be able to respond to the specific symptoms of the child, the personality and beliefs of the parents, and particular events that occur during the course of treatment. To enable this, the manual includes both a consistent sequence of treatment parts and flexible session modules. Eight *Parts* follow regularly in each case and are described in this chapter. Five *Session Modules* are detailed in the next chapter and are meant to be implemented by the therapist based on individual needs and events.

The Eight Parts of the Treatment

Part I Setting the Stage
Part II Charting Accommodation
Part III Choosing a Target Problem and Informing the Child
Part IV Formulating a Plan

Part V Reducing Accommodation—Continued
Part VI Additional Targets—Parents Take the Lead
Part VII Additional Targets—Continued
Part VIII Summary and Termination

The Five Session Modules

Session Module: Teaching the Child Anxiety Regulation Strategies
Session Module: Dealing with Extreme Disruptive Behavior
Session Module: Dealing with Threats of Self-Injury or Suicide
Session Module: Recruiting and Engaging Supporters
Session Module: Improving Collaboration Between Parents

PART I: SETTING THE STAGE

The purpose of the first part of the SPACE Program is to set the stage for the process that is to follow by defining overall goals for the treatment and creating a context for the work that is to come. Over the first one or two sessions the therapist has the four following goals:

1. Inform the parents that the intervention is aimed at *treating the child* although the means to do this is through work with the parents, and explain the rationale for parent work in anxiety.
2. Introduce the concept of *anxiety*.
3. Introduce the concept of the *personal boundary*.
4. Introduce the concept of *support*.

Introducing the Intervention

The first goals in treatment will be to establish a shared understanding of the program and its goals as well as to address possible worries or misconceptions parents may have about parent guidance. Then the therapist will introduce the core concepts and principles of the program before continuing to the active stages of behavioral change.

Why Parents?

Parent training or guidance almost inevitably raises certain questions in the minds of the parents who participate. Doubts such as: "Who is the patient here?"; "Are you saying this is my fault?"; "Why am I here when my child is the anxious one?" and others are valid and best addressed openly in a straightforward manner. The message conveyed to parents in the SPACE Program is that parents are participating primarily to help their child to better manage their anxiety and to prepare them for the future stressors they will face. The primary target of the treatment is the child's anxiety and ability to manage it. Although a successful course of treatment will likely improve parents' well-being and sense of competence, as well as freeing them from the need to accommodate the child's fear, the main goal is to treat the child's anxiety. It is important to stress this because unless parents understand that the treatment will actually benefit the child, it may not be prioritized highly enough to ensure their active participation in the therapy.

> I know you came to see me because of your child's anxiety and I want to clarify that that is exactly what we will be treating here. We are going to try to help her get much better at handling anxiety so that she will feel more comfortable in those situations that make her fearful or that she has been avoiding until now. In fact our goal is even more ambitious: Not only are we going to try to make her better at handling those situations — we are going to try to make her better at handling *any* anxiety. This is very important because when she has the tendency to be anxious, then even if she overcomes one fear, she may become anxious about something else soon after. By helping her to learn that she can handle anxiety in general, you can give her much more than you could by only teaching her that she doesn't don't need to fear this one thing. So that is our goal—to help her learn to cope much better with anxiety.

An important element of the SPACE Program is its focus on changing parent behavior as opposed to attempting to **directly** change the child's behavioral, cognitive, or emotional patterns. It is important for parents to understand that by changing their own behavior they can avoid much of the escalation that stems from trying to force their child to act differently. Additionally, as parents become more familiar with the interpersonal nature of anxiety in children (through the concepts of interpersonal boundaries and accommodation), it becomes more natural to view changes they make themselves as a means to changing the child as well.

Although we will be treating your child's anxiety, we know that just saying to someone who is afraid "Don't be afraid anymore," or "Do this and you will feel better about it," usually doesn't really work. As parents, you probably wish you could just flip some switch in your child's brain to make them think, act, or feel differently—but the truth is you can't. In fact, trying to make someone feel differently than they do usually makes them even more defensive. You may have already experienced this with your child?

Ask parents to describe prior attempts at directly changing child behavior, thought, or emotion and the results that this had. Discuss the reasons that this approach has not been successful and help parents to see that it is not because they have been "doing it wrong."

It is important that you understand that those attempts did not fail because you didn't think of the right thing to say, or because the wrong person said them. We simply can't *make* someone different, unless they ask us to help them change. That is why in this treatment we have something better. We have a tool so powerful that if we use it your child will almost certainly start to get better. And the wonderful thing is that this tool is one you actually *can* control. What is it? It is your own behavior! We know that if you can change your own behavior in some important ways then you can help your child to cope much better with anxiety!

Another issue that many parents will grapple with is the feeling of being blamed, criticized, or accused for the child's anxiety disorder. Even when parents initiate the parent guidance process or actively seek out parent training, they may still feel that by attempting to focus on their behavior rather than that of the child, the implicit message is "This is your fault." It is generally preferable to preempt this problem by openly stating that parent training does not mean that the problem is caused by the parents or that they are to blame. One way of stating this is to explain to parents: "You are not the problem here; however, you can be an important part of the solution." Some parents will benefit from an explanation that compares the parent work to the multitude of other ways in which parents help with children's issues, despite not being the "blame" for them:

Imagine that your child had a fever and was feeling sick. She was too sick to go to school and needed your help in getting to the doctor, taking medicine, or just some comfort to feel a little better. Would you feel that it was part of your job as a parent to help them? Of course you would. Might you need to act differently than on other days, for example, not insisting they go to school or perhaps even staying home yourself or checking in on them more often? You certainly might. Would it be your fault that they have the flu? Of course not! Blame is entirely irrelevant to the responsibility of parents to help their children overcome challenges and difficulties. It is part of what being a parent is all about. If your child is suffering from an anxiety disorder, you as a parent should do what you can to help them overcome it—this has nothing to do with blame! Sometimes, fulfilling that parental role means taking them to treatment and other times it means getting advice yourself. But either way, it is only about you being a mom or a dad.

Need for Active Steps and Hard Work Another important point the therapist will need to clarify in the early stages of treatment is that *coming to the sessions is not enough.* Attending weekly sessions with a skilled therapist may afford the parents a sense of support or empathy, and can provide them with a release valve for venting some of their frustration, but is unlikely to do much to alter the actual state of affairs for the child or in the home. In fact, the sense of being helped merely by talking about the problems can function as a perilous siren call in that, when the sessions are terminated as almost all therapeutic relationships eventually are, the parents may feel disappointed and conclude that parent-work is actually ineffective. Therefore, it is important to stress that the course of treatment will include, and indeed focus on, active steps that are planned together in the session and then implemented at home by the parents.

> Over the coming weeks I am going to suggest some steps that you can take at home to get the process of change going. We talk about these steps together here first, and it is important that you tell me about any doubts or questions that you have. Please be very open about any concerns you have, or if you don't agree with any of the ideas I suggest. Otherwise you probably won't feel comfortable actually doing these things at home. Keep in mind that I am knowledgeable about anxiety, but you have the most knowledge about **your child's** anxiety—so you will be able to offer insights that I couldn't have thought of. But also try to remember that

161

sometimes the things that seem most intuitive are actually not the best ones, or the most likely to work. After all, one reason you're coming here is because other things you tried didn't help enough. So please keep an open mind to new ideas and be willing to try things out. I can't promise you an easy process; in fact, this will probably be a lot of hard work! But remember that it is also a short treatment, so let's make this process a priority for the next couple of months. After all, when your child is feeling less anxious you may actually find that you have more time and energy because he needs less reassurance or because you are less worried.

Introduce the Concept of Unilateral Steps For many parents the biggest roadblock to successfully helping the child overcome anxiety is the belief that doing things in a unilateral way without the child's consent is wrong or contrary to their values. The therapist should address this value in a respectful way, but also highlight that when children are overly anxious they may need their parents to take initiatives that they are not yet capable of endorsing. By waiting interminably for the child to agree to work on the problem, they may be placing a burden on the children's shoulders that they are as yet incapable of bearing. Reframing unilateral parental action as a manifestation of concerned parenting and of leadership rather than as autarchic and dictatorial can help parents feel freer to act.

Most of the time, we prefer to solve every problem in a cooperative way. We believe in "talking things through" and "using our words" to resolve conflict, and in compromise as a way of managing interpersonal tensions. But all of these strategies rely on two sides working together and on a dialogue aimed at achieving common goals. Sometimes a child is just too anxious to be a partner in the process. In anxiety, just like in many other contexts, children often need their parents to guide them—even against their wishes. Many children actually secretly hope their parents will act without their agreement, because they understand that while something may seem frightening to them, doing nothing means not getting better. Think of your child as having many inner voices; some of the voices represent the fear and anxiety, and right now these may be clamoring the most loudly so that only they are heard. But consider that there are other voices inside as well. Voices that represent the child's will to be able to cope more, to be free to do more things or feel more comfortable. By acting independently of what the child is saying right now, you are aligning yourself with those voices and giving him or her your support.

Some children may feel compelled to resist the changes you make because of their anxiety. This is normal and to be expected. If children were able to take the long view and act in their own long-term best interests all the time, they wouldn't be children at all. They would be quite remarkable adults. However, it is important that you remind yourself that you are acting in your children's best interests and that the steps you take will not harm them. As we plan the steps you take, we will also talk about how to respond in a productive and supportive way to your child's reactions to the process.

What Is Anxiety?

At this point the therapist will provide the parents with information about anxiety, its function, and the ways it manifests in children. The goal here is not to create change by introducing this information but merely to create a common language on which to rely throughout the course of therapy, and to create a mutually shared framework on which to base the following steps.

Explain to parents that anxiety is the system all people have to alert them to danger, help them to avoid it and, when necessary, take steps to escape from it. Stress that anxiety is a healthy, necessary component of all children's psyche. Anxiety disorders exist when a child experiences exaggerated anxiety relating to things or situations that do not actually pose a real danger. For some children the anxiety system is triggered internally by worry, obsessive thoughts, or panic attacks, even when there are no external triggers for it. Children with anxiety disorders try to find ways to not experience anxiety, or to make themselves feel better when their anxiety is activated, just as other children do. The difference is that because of the disorder they need to do this more often or in less appropriate situations than other children.

Explain that anxiety includes behavioral, cognitive, emotional, and physiological aspects. Ask the parents to describe some of the ways in which each of these components is evident in their child's anxiety system. Explain that each of these components works in concert with the others, to form the full anxious response.

Introduce the Concept of Personal Boundary

The idea of the parental personal boundary, described later, can help parents to conceptualize the actions they will be taking over the course of treatment and provides a rationale for understanding them. Parents generally identify naturally with the idea that anxiety has made it harder for their child to function as independent individuals, has encroached on their own separateness, and has generally blurred the boundaries between themselves and their child. By emphasizing this process, the therapist helps parents to see their own reductions in accommodating to the anxiety as a means of restoring independence to the child rather than as self-serving or harsh. Additionally, reminding parents of the ways in which a child's anxiety affects the family system underlines the potential of parent work as a means of addressing the problem.

> As children grow they usually become more and more separated from their parents. They go different places, do different things, spend their time with other people, have different interests, and feel different emotions. However, because children rely on their parents when they are anxious, separation is difficult for a child with a lot of anxiety. It may be hard to spend time separately if your child is constantly worried about you, for example. Or if your children rely on you to do a lot of things instead of them, because they make them too nervous or uncomfortable it will be hard for them to function independently. This is natural and we refer to this as the effect that anxiety has on the *personal boundaries* separating child from parents.
>
> - Can you tell me about some ways in which your child's anxiety has impacted your personal boundaries?
> - Do you feel like your time is taken over by your child's fear? Do you do things your children would normally do for themselves?
> - Do you feel like your child is less independent than you would expect?
> - How does your child's anxiety affect you emotionally?
>
> You might say that one goal of this treatment is to create healthier boundaries so that your child can become more independent and more capable of handling things on his own.

Introduce the Concept of Parental Support

Explain that many parents who are faced with a child suffering from anxiety find themselves torn between two seemingly opposite poles. On the one hand, they may feel the need to reassure the child and help him or her to experience less anxiety. This may stem from empathy toward the children's distress or from a desire to help the children to function when anxiety is preventing them from doing so (for example, to help children go to school when they are anxious about that). On the other hand, many parents will also feel that by reassuring the child or accommodating to the anxiety they are not doing enough to promote the child's self-sufficiency. For many parents the opposing pulls of these two poles will result in an inconsistent fluctuation from a stance of over-protection to one that is overdemanding. Most often, what will determine the parents' specific reaction to any given situation will be arbitrary variables such as how tired or pressed for time they happen to be at that moment, rather than a clear plan of action.

If you are like most other parents of anxious children, you probably find yourself torn between the need to help your children feel better or get things done and the desire to show them that there is no real danger and that they can manage on their own. Being the parent of an anxious child usually means facing that dilemma thousands of times. What we have found is that, in fact, children respond the best when parents are able to combine both of those ideas into one message. In other words, the best reactions from parents to children's fears are those that combine an acceptance and legitimization of children's fears with a belief in that children's ability to withstand slightly more anxiety than they have until now. We call this combination *support*. When parents are only accepting the children's fear and reassuring them or helping them to avoid the anxiety, that is *protection*. When parents only expect their children to act bravely without recognizing the difficulty or accepting that the process may need to be gradual, we call that being *demanding*. But when parents are able to make children feel that they do understand and acknowledge how scared or uncomfortable they are, but they also steer them toward just a little more coping with the discomfort — that is *support*. In this treatment we will always look for ways for you to express that kind of support for your child.

- Discuss parents' thoughts about support.
- Ask whether parents feel they should accept the child's fear or should be trying to convince the child not to be afraid.

- Identify and address typical **demanding** statements/thoughts by parents such as:
  - It's not frightening.
  - I'm not afraid of it so it's fine.
  - Don't be a "wuss."
  - You're just acting like this for the attention.
- Identify and address typical **protection** statements/thoughts by parents such as:
  - She just can't handle stress.
  - Anxiety can hurt her/traumatize her/cause damage, and so on.
  - My job is to protect her from all this.
- Practice rephrasing *demanding* or *protection* statements into *support* statements, for example:

Instead of:

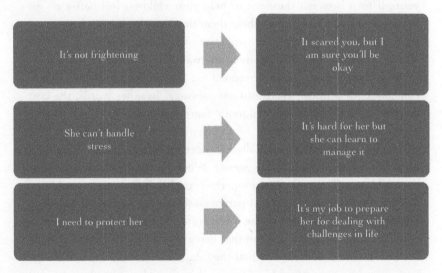

Demanding or overly protective statements can be rephrased to better reflect a supportive stance.

Intersession Goals

Ask both parents to write down one or two things that they would most like to see their child handling better. These may be things they have been avoiding or situations that make them overly uncomfortable or simply thoughts and questions they feel the child should not be thinking about.

PART II: CHARTING ACCOMMODATION

The goal of this session is to chart parent accommodation to child anxiety in detail. Accommodation can take various forms, such as parents adapting their schedule because of a child's anxiety, buying or providing items that the child requires because of anxiety, providing reassurance or answering questions triggered by anxiety, and performing actions on behalf of the child because of the child's avoidance.

The session has two parts:

1. Introducing the concept of accommodation and the reason to address it.
2. Charting accommodation for both parents.

Introducing Accommodation

Today I would like to talk with you about accommodation. Last time we talked about how anxiety affects the personal boundaries between parents and children. One thing that almost always will happen if your child is anxious is that she will rely on you for assistance in avoiding that anxiety. That's natural, and that's exactly what children are supposed to do when they feel threatened. The fact that your child relies on you shows us that she sees you as someone who cares and wants to help her, and that is a fine thing. Of course, one of our goals is to help her get better at *relying on herself,* but it's natural for her to have looked to you for protection until now.

Accommodation refers to any actions you may be doing, or even to things you are deliberately not doing, because of your child's anxiety disorder. Of course, helping a child to avoid things that are actually dangerous is not accommodation but rather healthy protection. So holding your child's hand when crossing the street, when they are too young to do it alone, is not accommodation but rather healthy protection. If your child is 16, however, and fully capable of crossing alone but afraid to do so, then holding his or her hand would be accommodation. You may be unsure about some of the things you are doing—are they accommodation or healthy protection? We can talk about these together.

Examples of Accommodation

There are endless possible ways in which parents may be accommodating children's anxiety symptoms. Below are some typical examples, but the therapist should be aware of the need for a thorough review of parental behavior relating to the anxiety.

- Speaking in place of a child with social anxiety.
- Sleeping next to a child who fears being in bed alone.
- Writing notes excusing a child from speaking in class or participating in other school behaviors.
- Not going out in the evening or only having one particular babysitter.
- Participating in OCD rituals such as hand washing or repetitive checking.
- Answering questions relating to a child's persistent worry.
- Providing the child with information about the parent's schedules or plans.
- Cutting food for a child who is afraid of touching a knife.
- Not inviting guests to the home.
- Not opening windows or shades.
- Not throwing away unnecessary items.
- Repetitive or overly rigid nighttime rituals.
- Reassuring a child they have not done wrong.
- Buying particular food products or avoiding specific foods because of a child's anxiety.
- Not bringing home books or movies with anxiety provoking stimuli.
- Driving particular routes.
- Refraining from using certain words.
- Swearing or promising that certain things will not happen.
- Taking a child to unnecessary medical checkups or procedures.

- Leaving lights on in the home.
- Not having balloons in the house.
- Preparing particular clothing articles.
- Doing homework instead of a child because of anxiety.
- Accompanying a child to a part of the house he or she fears approaching alone.

Charting Accommodation

Use the accommodation chart included later to create as detailed a description of the accommodating behaviors of both parents as possible, as well as any sibling accommodation. The chart should be completed with the therapist and should serve as a template, which can be changed and modified based on the needs and circumstances of the individual family and child.

When it is unclear whether a certain behavior is accommodation to anxiety or simply a parental choice, for example, the parent who chooses the child's clothing each day, or the parent who regularly telephones the child during the day to check up on him or her, try to use questions such as:

- Do (did) you do this with all your children?
- Would you like to be able to stop this behavior?
- If your child were not anxious would you still do this?
- What would happen if you did not do this one day?

Behaviors that express the parents' protection (or overprotection) of the children, but do not serve to alleviate the children's anxiety or to help them to avoid, should not be included in this chart but should be noted separately. For example, if a parent changes the sheets on a child's bed each night because *the parent* has a contamination-related fear, this should not be included in the accommodation chart but is important information. Similarly, the parent who does not allow a child to participate in sleepovers is not accommodating to child anxiety but may be overly protective of the child.

Accommodation Chart			
List all forms of accommodation for each part of the day. Describe briefly the change in parent or sibling behavior prompted by the child's anxiety. Specify if accommodation recurs regularly.			
	Father	Mother	Siblings
Morning			
Getting up			
Getting dressed			
Breakfast			
Going to school			
Other			
School/work			
Afternoon			
Pick up from school			
Lunch			
Homework			
Out-of-school activities			
Social activities			
Other			
Evening			
Supper			
"Family time"			
Prebedtime			
Other			
Bedtime			
Getting ready for bed			

Washing up/showering			
Going to bed			
Other:			
Nighttime			
Weekend			
Other			
Other			

Intersession Goals

- Ask parents to continue charting accommodation each day, using the accommodation chart over the course of the coming week until the next session.
- Ask parents to choose one target accommodation-related behavior that they feel most limits the child's independence or most interferes with their own routine, and which they would like to address in treatment.

Try to think of one thing each about which you can say to yourself: "If we can make that one thing better I will be glad we came here." Of course, we will probably address more things as we go, but try to pick the one that seems the very most important to you right now.

CONSIDER SESSION MODULES

- Teaching the child anxiety regulation strategies.
- Recruiting and engaging supporters.

PART III: CHOOSING A TARGET PROBLEM AND INFORMING THE CHILD

This session has two parts:

1. Choosing a target problem.
2. Planning to inform the child of the parent-led process.

171

Choosing a Target Problem

At the beginning of the session the therapist reviews the intersession goals with the parents. This includes updating the accommodation chart with new information the parents provide and asking parents about the target problem they chose as most important. In the event that one or both of the parents did not give this adequate thought or had difficulty making a decision at home, ask them to try to indicate now what they feel would be the most important goal.

Based on the answers of both parents, and on the criteria described later for adequate target problems, the therapist will try to agree with the parents on the problem to be addressed first. A good target problem will have the following characteristics:

- **It will be accommodation-oriented**—In other words, it will be a problem in which the parents are involved through their accommodating behaviors. For example, some parents may indicate a child's refusal to speak in the classroom as the biggest problem. This, however, is not an ideal first target (although it can become a target at a later stage), because the parents are likely not actively involved in that situation. In contrast, a related but different problem such as the need to speak in place of the child in various situations would be accommodation-oriented.

- **It will be a "significant problem"**—This is a subjective definition based primarily on parental opinion and assessment. For example, some parents may feel that a child sleeping in their bed every night is a significant problem while others may feel it is merely a small inconvenience or even a normative behavior. Most significant problems will be those that impact either a child's ability to function in day-to-day life in appropriate ways, or that impact significantly on parents' ability to pursue their own routines and agendas. One phone call a day to a parent's workplace may not create a significant problem, but 10 calls in a day may interfere with the workday tremendously.

- **It will be a recurrent problem**—This refers to the frequency with which the problematic situation recurs in the life of the family. For example, some parents may indicate a child's inability to fly on airplanes as the biggest problem because it means not being able to

172

take the vacation they want. However, this would not be a suitable problem because the frequency is so low. On the other hand, not being able to drive in a car because of a fear of becoming carsick may create a frequently recurring issue.

- **It will be one that parents are motivated to address** — This point is particularly important because, as parents begin taking the active steps necessary to create change, their motivation is likely to be tested. The less determined they are at the outset of the process, the more likely they are to abandon it before the goal has been achieved. For this reason the best target problem is one that the parents see as being a "no choice" situation. In other words, they feel as though they absolutely must address this issue because it is vital to the welfare or future of themselves or their child.
- **Avoid nonanxiety-related problems** — Anxiety is a construct used broadly and it is easy for parents in the treatment process to feel motivated at a given moment by problems that do not stem directly from the anxiety disorder. Children who do not clean their room *may* be exhibiting compulsive hoarding behavior, but the issue could also be less closely anxiety-related.

It is helpful to clarify to parents that the first target problem chosen does not have to be the last one. In fact it is likely that there will be additional targets addressed over the course of treatment, or even after treatment concludes, by the parents themselves, using the skills and strategies learned. However, attempting to correct everything at once or undertaking too many goals at the same time will most often lead to none of them being accomplished. Conversely, succeeding at even one goal will make undertaking additional goals easier in the future. In addition, many children will display independent improvement in additional spheres as they learn that they are capable of overcoming anxiety.

I know that there are other problems that you are also hoping to work on and that this problem is not the only one on your plate. You probably want to ask "Well, what should we do about that other thing while we are working on this?" I am going to advise you to keep doing what you have been doing for the time being. And make a conscious choice not to argue about it between yourselves or with your child. If we try to fight all battles at once we will almost certainly spread ourselves much too thinly. Remember that by making even one small change you are teaching your child a tremendously important lesson—that they can get better. And that you can help them to do it. Once they have learned that, it will be easier to get better at another thing as well. It will be difficult enough for your child to make this one change; we can't expect him to tackle everything else at the same time. But often, even without us saying anything at all, children start improving at other anxiety-related issues. This tells us they are beginning to see themselves as much stronger.

Informing the Child

The point at which parents inform the child of their determination to generate a process of change in the target problem is an important and pivotal one. Children may respond to the parents' message in any number of ways. Some will express interest, curiosity, or even enthusiasm. Others will exhibit indifference. Children whose anxiety is triggered by the parents' intentions may respond more negatively; many become angry or argumentative, querying the parents' precise plans or attempting to draw them into lengthy debates over the wisdom of their intents. Others may react with hostility and yet others will exhibit dramatic displays of distress that parents may find difficult to withstand.

Explain to the parents that although it is important to make clear to the children that they are a welcome and important part of the process, it is best not to confuse this with a debate over whether the process will happen. Parents who confuse this issue will generate corresponding doubt in the mind of the child, and will unintentionally encourage more debate and ensuing argument than parents who stick to a "This is our decision, and we hope you are willing to work with us" style of presentation. In many cases the two parents will have, in the past, represented markedly different attitudes to the child's anxiety and the child may have correspondingly different behavior with each parent. Therefore, it is important that both parents be present when informing the child of the plan. In this way the unspoken message is clear: "We agree about this and have decided on it together."

Find a time when you and your child are both calm and relaxed. It is important to have both of you present for this discussion, so make sure to pick a time when you are both free of other obligations and distractions. You may need to arrange for someone to watch the other siblings while you are having this conversation, or perhaps choose a time when they are out of the home. This part of the process should never be done at the moment at which your child's anxiety has been triggered. In other words, if your child is afraid of going down into the basement alone and has just come up after a failed attempt to go there, don't take that moment as the opportunity to say "You know, we really need to talk about that—we are going to be working on that very fear." Rather, wait for a time when your child is not acting fearful and you are not feeling frustrated by his avoidance.

Sit down with him in a relaxed way and say, "We know how difficult it is for you to do _____ (fill in as appropriate). We understand it makes you feel really anxious or afraid. We want you to know that this is perfectly natural and everyone feels afraid some of the time. But we also want you to know that it is our job as your parents to help you get better at things that are hard for you, and we have decided to do exactly that. We are going to be working on this for a while and we know it will probably take time, but we love you too much not to help you when you need help. Soon we'll talk about it again and we will have some ideas for things to do that will make you get better at handling _____. We are really very proud of you!"

Dealing with Resistance — The Written Announcement

In many cases parents have already tried to discuss the anxiety with the child often in the past and have been met with resistance or even outbursts of anger at raising the issue. This merely reflects the acute anxiety that the child experiences at the idea of attempting to overcome the fear, and is best thought of as a sign of distress rather than as misbehavior. Nevertheless, attempting to repeat the same experience once again is likely to exacerbate the negative behavior, and can also seem like a daunting proposition for the parents to undertake. In this situation or in other cases where communication between the parents and the anxious child had become difficult or explosive, we recommend replacing the spoken communication with a written announcement. The four purposes of the written announcement are:

1. To inform the child of the parents' intent without inviting escalation.
2. To practice unilateral action on the part of the parents—a key to future success.
3. To create parental commitment and adherence to the process.
4. To allow the parents to express their message precisely and concisely.

The text of the announcement should reflect the following principles, as exemplified in the sample announcements below.

The Announcement Is Empathic and Supportive An empathic announcement that explicitly acknowledges the child's difficulty realizes the principle of support by combining empathy with a determination to overcome the difficulty, and a commitment to change. By starting the announcement with an empathic statement, the parents make it clear that their acts are not based on indifference to the child's inner world, and do not reflect an attitude of blame or criticism. Many parents feel that any determination on their part is equal to an accusation against the child, as though by saying "We believe you can do better" they are implying "You should have already been doing better." In fact, often parents react to the idea of expecting the child to overcome the anxiety with comments such as "But he's really a good kid!," or "It's not his fault!," or "He's already suffering enough!" Beginning the announcement with expressions of empathy shows the parents' compassion for the child, even as they are determined to battle the anxiety.

The Announcement Focuses on the Parents The aim of the announcement is to clearly express the parents' attitude and beliefs; for that reason it centers on them—their thoughts, their feelings, and their plans. An announcement centered on the child, such as, "From now on you will . . . " or "As of today you may not . . . " leads to arguments and resistance. Focusing on the children may cause them to feel they need to prove to the parents that they are wrong, and that they cannot force them to change. An announcement that focuses on the parents' intentions concedes that they can only control their side of the relationship

176

with their child. This emphasis reinforces their personal boundary; the message delivered is: "This is our position, but we cannot dictate your reaction!"

A Clear and Concrete Announcement   One guaranteed way of confusing a clear message is to bury it under a mountain of vague statements. For example: "From now on we expect you to act your age!" or "We will act to ensure you live a normal life!" or even a well-intentioned "You need to become more able to manage anxiety." Statements such as these resemble a lecture more than a clear announcement. The announcement should focus directly on the target problem that has been agreed on. Although a focused statement describes a clear boundary, a blurry one is actually an invitation to examination, experimentation, and breach.

The Announcement Includes a Notice About the Involvement of Supporters from Outside the Home   Enlisting the support of others, from outside the immediate nuclear family, is a tremendous source of strength and an effective way of minimizing escalation. As detailed in subsequent sessions and session modules, this is a keystone to creating and preserving momentum in otherwise stagnant situations. Including this in the announcement makes it easier for the parents to implement this tool in the coming weeks. The announcement should therefore include the statement that the parents "will turn to any person who can offer them support and help them in the process." Parents should make it clear that their aim is not to embarrass the child, but to help in overcoming the problem.

Presenting the Announcement
The same principles apply to presenting the written announcement as to verbally informing the child of the parents' plan to work on the problem. In other words, it should be done with both parents present and involved, at a time when parents and child are relaxed and never as an immediate response to the child's anxiety-triggered avoidance. In one extreme example of diverging from these principles, a father waited for his daughter to (predictably) refuse to enter a social event because of social anxiety and then pounced on her with a loud "Aha!" while

whipping the announcement out of his back pocket! Wisely choosing a more relaxed time will invariably lead to better results.

> Find a time when your child is relaxed, perhaps while reading or listening to music, or watching TV in his room, and then enter the room together. Focus him on you by sitting down calmly, and when you have his attention say simply, "There is something we have been thinking about and need to tell you. Because it was so important to us that we say just what we meant, we decided to write it down." Read the announcement aloud and then hand him the written letter or place it next to him. At this point the best thing is to leave the child to his thoughts and avoid discussing the content of the letter.

Sample Announcement I—An 11-Year-Old Girl with Separation Anxiety

> Ashley, we know that you suffer greatly every time you have to stay home alone, and at bedtime. We see how hard these moments are for you, and how much your fears are hurting you. But we also realize that our behavior so far, staying with you constantly, and allowing you to sleep with us in our bed, not only didn't help, but actually made things worse. Therefore, we have decided that from now on we will no longer ignore the problem. We will help you not give in to your fears. We will talk with you again soon about some changes, such as us going out more and helping you to stay in your own bed. We have also decided not to keep the problem a secret. We are proud of you and we will turn to anyone we think of who can help us. We will gladly give you all the support you need to deal with your fears, including therapy, if you want it. But the support will not be by giving in to your fears. —Your loving parents.

Sample Announcement II—A 9-Year-Old Boy with School Phobia and Refusal

> Steven, we love you so much. We understand that going to school, and even thinking about it, makes you very uncomfortable. We saw how hard you tried to go and we know you are truly anxious about it. We also believe that going to school is extremely important for you and we are completely confident that you will able to overcome this fear. We have decided not to allow you to stay home from school anymore and we will be doing everything we can to make sure that this changes. We are not angry at you and are not trying to punish you. We simply care too much

to allow your fear to hurt you in this way. We will be getting help from anyone who can help us to succeed at this challenge and we hope you will work together with us on this problem. We love you very much — Mom and Dad.

Sample Announcement III — A 14-Year-Old Boy with Compulsive Showering

Adam, we love you very much and think you are a wonderful boy. We know how uncomfortable you have been feeling recently and how OCD can make you think you are not clean enough and need to shower for hours every day. We realize it is a very difficult thing for you to ignore. But we are your parents and it is our job to help you with problems. We are sure you are strong enough to win against OCD and we have decided it is our job to help you do that. We will do our best from now on to make sure that OCD cannot make you take such long showers because this is interfering with your life. We know if you could simply choose to stop right away you would, and we do not blame you for this problem. We simply have decided to do our job in helping you get better. We also plan to get as much help as we can in fighting OCD and will be talking about this problem with anyone we believe can help. Together we are sure we can do this. With love, Mom and Dad.*

Dealing with Parental Reactions to the Announcement

Many parents are apprehensive about creating and presenting their child with a written announcement in this way and it is helpful to discuss any misgivings in the session, before the actual announcement.

Why So Formal?   Although the formal nature of a written announcement may seem strange, stilted, or even distasteful to some parents who prefer a more natural and spontaneous form of communication, it is actually the formality itself that provides some important benefits. By acting in a way that is clearly different from what usually happens, the parents are indicating, to both themselves and the child, that this is a

---

*In this announcement the parents take pains to externalize the obsessive-compulsive disorder as a separate entity rather than as their son's will — allowing them to portray themselves as allied with him against a common "enemy" rather than as resisting his will.

turning point; that things will be different from before. This is an important message, as most parents will have already had many unfruitful "natural" conversations in the past that did not lead to change. Formality adds a ceremonious feel to the situation that conveys a sense of importance and solemnity, thereby amplifying the impact of the message. The child feels that the parents have put thought into the matter and this expresses a caring that is meaningful to their experience.

Why in Writing? Because that way you will say what you meant to say! There is simply no way around it: When the message is not written down the chances are good that parents will end up saying much more than they planned, and probably quite different things. Without a written text they are more likely to be sidetracked by interruptions from the child or distracted by divergent trains of thought as in:

> "Son we love you very much and . . . "
>
> "No you don't!"
>
> "Of course we do, why would you say that!?"
>
> . . . And so on.

Additionally, when parents rely on their own improvisation rather than a prepared text they will most likely say or emphasize the things that come most naturally to them (or to whichever parent does the actual talking). In this scenario, important parts of the announcement that do not feel as natural or intuitive may be left out or underemphasized. For example, the announcement included a clear acknowledgment that the child is actually afraid. For many children the written announcement will be the first time they ever hear their parents openly admit this—something that may end up missing from a less structured or carefully scripted text.

She Won't Listen to Us This parental reaction is clearly indicative of long-standing frustration in the relationship and of a need for supplying the parents with tools to effectively communicate with their child. The written announcement is just such a tool. The best response to this is "It doesn't matter." The parents' job is merely to make the announcement— not to shape the child's reaction:

You do not need to make her listen. Simply enter the room and try to draw her attention. If she chooses to ignore you, just go ahead with the announcement. Remember that even if she seems to be ignoring you she's most likely paying close attention. If she puts on her earphones or picks up a book don't react to this. It will only serve to make you feel less effective. Just read the announcement, place it next to her, and leave the room. If you did what you planned to do you were successful — no matter what she did!

It Won't Help   Of course it won't! The purpose of the announcement is not to change the behavior or to solve the problem. It is merely to inform the child in a clear and resolute way of the plan to address the issue. There is no expectation that it will "help" in any immediate sense.

Dealing with Child Reactions to the Announcement

Children react to the announcement in many different ways, most of which can be grouped into the following categories. Role-play with the parents the recommended responses to the various forms of resistance.

Argument, Debate, and Emotional Blackmail   In this category we include all verbal responses that attempt to convince the parents not to pursue this plan. Some children will try to explain that they are "really afraid," something the parents have already acknowledged in the text of the announcement. Others may say, and believe, that trying to make them face the fear will only make it much worse. Some might attempt to bargain for more time ("Next school year I promise to be back to normal") while others will query the specific intents of the parents ("What exactly are you going to do?"). Many children will focus on the element of including others in the situation and beg their parents to respect their privacy by not doing so.

The best response to this kind of argument and debate is one of not agreeing to engage in it. Parents should simply say one time to the child, in a calm and quiet voice: "We have told you what we meant to say and now we will be thinking about what to do next. We are not going to talk about this anymore right now." By saying this one time and then refusing to answer additional argumentative comments or questions, children will eventually stop on their own accord, and the parental message will be preserved.

On the other hand, engaging in argument or attempting to convince children that they are acting correctly will almost certainly detract from both the clarity of the message and from their own inner resolve.

Another reaction, which is particularly trying to parents, is that of emotional blackmail. By this we refer to statements such as, "If you loved me you would not do this to me," or similar claims. It is helpful to prepare parents in advance for this possibility as it is clearly hard not to become drawn into this dynamic.

> You know in your heart and your belly that you love this child and that you are acting out of love for her. This is not the time to try to prove that or to convince her of the fact. Sometimes children will feel that way, and more commonly they will say it because they recognize the impact it has on you. By overcoming the emotional discomfort this kind of statement causes you—you are actually expressing your love in the most important way! You are allowing yourself to be hurt **because** you love her so much.

Another form of emotional blackmail includes threats by the child to themselves, such as the threat of running away or the threat of self-harm or suicide. Although these threats are not infrequent they do not generally imply an immediate concern for the child's safety. Nevertheless, suicidal threats should never be taken lightly by parents or clinicians and we provide guidance on dealing with them in a separate session module devoted specifically to this anxiety-provoking topic.

Indifference, Ignoring, and Scorn   Another frequently reported category of reactions include all the ways in which a child may verbally or otherwise convey to the parents the message: "I don't care what you think or say." These include things like refusing to face the parents or to make eye contact, hiding under a blanket, feigning sleep, or even more childish forms such as sticking their fingers in their ears and saying "I can't hear you." Although children may work hard to convey indifference, this is usually precisely because they are apprehensive about the parents' plans, or emotionally moved by the content of the announcement. Nevertheless, it is invariably unhelpful to reflect this to the children or to insist on their attention.

By deciding what you want to say and saying it, you are taking control of the situation. You are "driving" your own behavior. When you insist that your child pay attention to you, you are relinquishing this control and putting them in charge. You may feel like you are being authoritative by yelling, "You need to listen to me" but, in fact, you are actually saying "I need you to listen and don't know how to handle the fact that you won't; until you do I am stuck!"

In other words, parents should carry out their plan regardless of the child's attention or respect. An attempt should be made at the start to focus attention on the parents, and most often simply entering the room, or sitting down, will be enough. If the child displays ignoring behavior the parents should make a single additional attempt by saying: "There is something we want to say to you, could you listen now?" or "Please turn off the TV, we need to talk with you." If the ignoring continues, parents should proceed nonetheless without additional insistence on the child's attention. We recommend that parents not turn off the television the child is watching and more importantly not attempt to physically direct the child to themselves (as in yanking earphones out of the child's ears), as this will likely escalate the situation rapidly and can lead to disruptive or explosive behavior. One form of ignoring is particularly confusing to parents despite being very basic—the child leaves the room before the announcement is complete. In this case, too, if the child is within hearing range, the parents should complete the announcement and place it on the child's desk or bed, and leave the room without further discussing the issue. If the child is not within hearing range, they should leave the written announcement for the child and avoid discussing the matter.

Some children may exhibit scorn toward the parents, for example, by mocking or imitating them or by means of other disparaging gestures. Here, too, parents should make every effort to continue unperturbed with their original plan and not be distracted by a need to discipline the child. For some parents it may be helpful to reframe this behavior as an anxiety-provoked defensive mechanism rather than an undisciplined lack of respect that requires correcting. In other cases it may be most helpful to remind the parents that a child's provocative behavior is an attempt to distract them from their purpose of addressing the anxiety. Therefore, if the focus of the conversation shifts away from the anxiety and on to the disrespectful behavior, the parents are actually rewarding the behavior rather than discouraging it.

Another form of scorn we have encountered frequently entails the child tearing up the announcement or crumpling it into a ball and even throwing it at the parents. This, too, should be ignored, but parents may find comfort that, in our experience, many children later retrieve the disgraced letter and keep it; some of them even cherish it in secret. This reflects the duality of inner voices described earlier, in which children are compelled to resist coping because of their fear but simultaneously hoping for someone to help them get better.

Aggressive Behavior   This category can include anything from yelling at the parents to leave the room or other verbal abuse, to threats directed at the parents, and even to actual acts of violence. Once again it is important to remember that these behaviors likely represent the strong anxiety the child is feeling. When possible, parents should be advised to ignore the behavior and to make the announcement, leave the written letter, and quietly exit the room without reacting to the aggression. This is appropriate for verbal aggression, including threats and for mild physical behaviors, such as tossing a pillow toward the parents. When a child becomes more aggressive (i.e., hitting, kicking), parents should simply leave the written announcement and exit the room. We recommend not addressing this behavior in this instance although in later sessions parents will be introduced to means of reacting effectively to aggressive behavior in non-escalatory ways.

Distress   In this category we include reactions that involve displays of distress such as crying or sobbing dramatically. These displays usually reflect true distress but can also be a means of putting pressure on the parents to reassure them that they will not do anything unpleasant or difficult. For obvious reasons parents will have to resist this impulse, despite the emotional stress of doing so. Once the announcement has been completed, parents can comfort children by hugging them or otherwise soothing them but should refrain from talking about the content of the announcement itself. Questions about the anxiety should be avoided and, as with the more argumentative child, parents should state clearly one time that they are considering how best to act and will not discuss it further at this point.

Intersession Goals

Following this session the parents proceed to inform the child. It is usually advisable for them to do this one or two days before the next session, to avoid a lengthy time between the announcement and the steps that follow. Ask parents to reflect on their feelings before, during, and after the actual announcement (i.e., apprehension, dread, resolve, optimism, helplessness, competence, hope).

CONSIDER SESSION MODULES

- Teaching the child anxiety regulation strategies.
- Recruiting and engaging supporters.
- Improving collaboration between parents.

PART IV: FORMULATING A PLAN

The goal of this session is to follow up on informing the child (verbally or by means of a written announcement) by planning clear behavioral changes that the parents will make to their behavior. These will be closely tied to the target problem chosen earlier and of which the child was informed. The changes will usually involve the reduction of accommodating behaviors on the part of the parents but can also include steps taken by the parents to resist the avoidance on the part of the child.

Review of Announcement

Therapist and parents review the act of informing the child. The review should address both the factual and emotional components of the experience. Factual elements include the time and place, what was said, and the child's behavior. Parents' emotional experience is also experience and may include a sense of success, failure, disappointment, or potentially conflict between the two parents. Stress the idea that regardless of the child's response—if the parents made the announcement they have successfully completed an important step.

Reducing Accommodating Behaviors

This process is usually done in a gradual way with specific guidelines for what accommodation will continue and what will be changed. The therapist should work with the parents to ensure that both parents are clear about the behavioral changes and agree to them. Often one parent will need help in expressing a point of view and ensuring it is a factor in the process, and it is important that the therapist be alert to this possibility.

Examples of Plans for Reducing Accommodation for a Child with Repeated Phone Calls to Parents Throughout the Day

- Mother and father will each not respond to more than one phone call a day.
- Mother and father will each call child one time per day. Mother will call at 2 P.M. and father will call at 4 P.M.
- Child will be rewarded—one Disney princess card—for every day they do not call each parent more than one time.
- Child will be informed of this in advance.
- Child will be instructed to send a text message in case of urgent need to communicate with parents. The text message must include the specific reason for calling. Any other messages will not be responded to.

For a Child Who Insists Parents Participate in Washing Rituals

- Parents will not wash their hands in the child's presence (will wash normally—alone).
- Parents will not answer any questions regarding their hand washing.
- Parents will not allow child to "inspect" their hands.
- Child will be informed in advance of the changes to parent behavior, including a clear statement that parents will maintain cleanliness as they see fit.

Part IV: Formulating a Plan

For a Child with Separation Anxiety Who Will Not Stay Alone

- Parents will leave the home together for 5 minutes each evening—time to be increased gradually.*
- Parents will take their phone but will not respond to calls from child.*
- Parents will arrange for another person (possibly aunt or uncle) to speak on the phone with child while parents are out of the house—if child wishes.
- Child will be informed of the plan in detail—including exact time that parents will be out.
- Parents will be careful to return after specified time.

For a Child Who Insists on Sealed Windows and Does Not Allow Strangers in the Home or Changes to Home

- Parents will open the window in their room including blinds—to be followed by additional windows in the house.
- Parents will invite at least three guests to the home over the coming week. Guests may address child and speak with him, but will not enter child's room unless invited.
- Parents will make one significant change to shared home space (either new rug in living room or new arrangement of seating—to be decided by parents).
- Changes to the home will be done while child is out or in his room—to avoid escalation.

For a Child with Extended "Good Night Rituals" Involving Both Parents

- One parent will say good night to child in bed—the other will say good night in the living room.
- Parent will leave the room immediately after saying good night.
- Parent will return to room after 20 minutes if child is awake or in distress but will not perform ritual. Parent will say "I know you are feeling uncomfortable right now, but I'm sure you will be okay."

---

*If child is willing to engage in the process then the length of parents' absence and the issue of responding to the phone will be negotiable. If child refuses to collaborate then parents will leave for the planned 5 minutes and not answer the phone.

- Child will not be punished for staying up or acting out unless there is physical aggression.
- In the morning both parents will say, "I'm proud of you—you got to sleep without the rituals."
- If child becomes overly distressed for more than 1 hour then the following night parents will arrange for aunt to stay in the home and will leave the house after saying good night once. .
- Child will be informed of the plan—apart from the possibility of parents leaving the home.

Informing the Child

Most of the principles described in the context of informing the child about the intent to address the anxiety disorder will apply to informing them about the specific changes as well. Namely, the parents should present their decision in a quiet, supportive way that emphasizes their understanding of the difficulty for the child as well as their confidence in her ability to cope. Below is an example of informing the child of the plan described above for a girl with repeated phone calls throughout the day:

> Monica, last week we told you we were going to be thinking about ways to help you get better at handling the worry-thoughts you have every day. We know those thoughts make you really scared and are proud of you for doing so well at school and dance despite the thoughts. Even though you think you really need to talk to us on the phone when you have those thoughts, we are sure that you will actually be okay even if you don't talk to us. We believe that 100%. That's why from now on Mom and Dad are not going to answer the phone when you call us at work more than one time. You can talk to each of us one time and after that we will not answer any more. Because we know how hard it might be for you, we will also call you one time every day. Mom will call you at 2 and Dad will call you at 4. When you manage not to call each of us more than one time you will get a prize—one Disney princess card. If it is too hard for you one day and you call us more often than one time you can always try again the next day. But even if you do call we will not answer after the first time. If you have something that is really urgent to

tell us, you can send mom or dad a text message and tell us what the matter is. We will decide if we should call you or not. We know this could be hard and we are not trying to punish you or hurt you. We love you and want to help.

When a child has responded positively to the original announcement, the new information should be presented in as collaborative a way as possible. In other words, parents should describe the plan as a joint effort by parents and child to overcome anxiety. Whenever possible the child can, and should, be invited to take part in planning the details of the plan. In the case of the child with separation anxiety earlier, for instance, the child was invited to determine the length of the parents' departure from the home. In essence, when the child agrees to cooperate they should be given as much control as possible over the process. This will help to maintain motivation and reduce conflict. However, the conversation should be limited to the details of the plan and parents should refuse to engage in debate over the core concept of gradually overcoming the anxiety.

When the child has responded negatively to the announcement, or when communication around the anxiety issue (or in general) is particularly strained, the parents should employ a more unilateral approach. Parents should write the plan and present it in a manner similar to the written announcement described in the previous session. In this way, if they are not able to speak with the children about it they can still provide them with the pertinent information by leaving the written note for them to see.

Dealing with Child Reactions to Decreased Accommodation

Reducing accommodation will almost inevitably increase the child's anxiety in the short term, and parents need to be prepared for this both emotionally and practically, in terms of responses to child behavior. Discussing the parents' thoughts or fears regarding the way their child will react and role playing those situations together can be helpful in creating confidence about their ability to persevere despite potential stress.

Keep in mind that we are changing the rules that the child has come to rely on and to which you have conformed for a long time. It took a long time for you to feel prepared to take action to overcome the anxiety and it is unrealistic to expect your child to feel just as prepared simply because you decided to act. You are doing what you know to be necessary and helpful in the long run, but your child may not see it that way yet and we cannot expect her to. Be prepared for her to feel more anxious or even to feel a sense of betrayal at your decisions. And remember that right now she needs you to be strong for her because she is not yet ready to be strong for herself. Sometimes being a parent is about doing what's right for your child even when they don't want you to.

Disengagement
Although some children may respond in dramatic or challenging ways, parents should learn the most important rule:

The less you respond, the more quickly the emotion will subside!

This rule holds true for many different kinds of emotional outbursts a child might exhibit. For example, children who feel a need to have a reassurance-seeking question answered may follow their parents around the house for a long time repeating the question and begging to have it answered. This is tremendously difficult to ignore. However, parents who successfully remain disengaged and do not become drawn in to the interaction will see their child more quickly distracted by another thought or simply exhausted by the persistent repetition. In contrast, children whose parents continue to engage with them around the issue (for example, "I said I would not answer that"; "It's not that I don't want to, it's that I think you can be okay," or simply "Leave me alone") will continue the process for much longer. The simple rule that every child knows is: *As long as we are talking about this—there's a chance you'll change your mind!*

Distancing
When a child's reactions are particularly explosive, the parents should attempt to actually distance themselves from the child until he or she is calm again. Rather than responding to the behavior itself or attempting to correct it, parents should simply walk away, perhaps

going to their room or even leaving the house for a while (when this is safely possible).

Presence of Supporters

One reliable way to reduce the level of drama created by the change in the parent's behavior is to have other people present in the home when these changes are implemented. Although most actions parents take to actively subdue a child's outbursts will have the opposite effect, the presence of additional people can be extremely helpful. Such a presence will almost invariably inhibit the most problematic behaviors a child may otherwise exhibit, such as physical aggression or violence toward property. Physical violence as a means of enforcing accommodation is common, although little discussed, and should be considered as a potential result of the parents' steps.

- When parents foresee explosive behavior from the child in response to their actions, the presence of supporters should always be part of the plan. See the session module devoted specifically to this for details on recruiting and utilizing supporters before directing parents to take the accommodation-reducing steps.
- The therapist should make every effort to be available to the parents (i.e., email, telephone) between sessions for the coming weeks, during which parents begin to modify their behavior. This will allow more rapid addressing of difficulties and create a stronger sense of support. Parents should be encouraged to utilize this increased accessibility.

Intersession Goals

The parents take the following three steps following this session:

1. Informing the child.
2. Implementing the plan formulated in the session.
3. Charting accommodation—for the target problem. Parents should try to adhere successfully to the plan 100% of the time, but should not be expected to be totally successful. They should monitor their successes and setbacks as well as the child's reactions.

CONSIDER SESSION MODULES

- Recruiting and engaging supporters.
- Improving collaboration between parents.
- Dealing with extreme disruptive behavior.
- Dealing with threats of self-injury or suicide.
- Teaching the child anxiety regulation strategies.

PART V: REDUCING ACCOMMODATION—CONTINUED

The following sessions focus on implementing, monitoring, and gradually developing the plan to reduce parental accommodation to the child's anxiety. Throughout the sessions the therapist should implement the Session Modules based on individual needs and developments. Each Session Module includes guidelines for the therapist as an aid in determining when to include them in the process.

Review of the Past Week

Begin the session with a review of the week that has gone by, guiding parents to address each of the following aspects of the week.

Parents' Success at Reducing Their Own Accommodation

Discuss the situations in which parents felt most successful and effective at modifying their accommodating behaviors, and those in which they found it most difficult or were not able to do so. An exclusive focus on the most problematic situations can create a sense of discouragement, which will lower motivation. Strive to maintain a balance between positive and negative experiences. Avoid recrimination, including criticisms from the therapist, self-blame, and accusatory remarks from one parent to the other, such as, "I did what we planned, and you undermined me."

Child's Reactions to the Changes

Discuss the ways in which the child reacted to the steps the parents have taken over the week. Child reactions include not only the immediate reaction such as when the parents refuse to accommodate but also behaviors that follow later and seem to relate to the parental decisions. For instance, many children react negatively in the moment but later seem more relaxed than usual. Other children will act in a negative way at first but later apologize or seek to spend time with the parents in a positive way. Ask parents to describe any additional changes they have witnessed in the child over the week that deviate from existing behavioral patterns.

It is useful to compare the changes in the child's reactions over repeated instances of the same parental step. For example, children may cry for more than an hour the first time their parents refuse to engage in a compulsive ritual but only cry for 15 minutes the third time. Although both these instances will pose a stressful event for the parents, the change can demonstrate a growing capacity for self-regulation on the part of the child.

- Specifically ask about any extremely troubling or dangerous reactions the child may have exhibited, such as physical violence, acts or threats of self-injury, or other extreme behaviors. See the Session Module on dealing with threats of self-injury if necessary.

Reinforce Progress

Small changes can easily be disregarded or overlooked in the context of everything that goes on in a family's life in one week. However, reflecting these small steps to parents can make a big difference to their ability to persevere. Additionally, parents who themselves are not focusing on the progress a child is making are also not likely to be reinforcing the change in the child. Help parents to identify even small improvements and encourage them to reflect these to the child in the form of praise.

Parental Change Is Progress

Some parents become overly focused on the change they hope to see in the child's behavior and miss an important point. Just by successfully changing their own behavior they are already making progress—no matter how the child reacted. This is particularly true in the context of accommodation reduction because if they successfully declined to accommodate, parents have already done at least three important things:

1. They have shown themselves and the child that they can make a plan and enact it.
2. They have conveyed a clear message to the child that they are confident in his or her ability to withstand the anxiety.
3. By reducing the accommodation they have led the child to find alternative ways to overcome the anxiety.

When Monica's parents returned to the next session they seemed disheartened. "It's not helping" was their sentiment. In reviewing the past week it became apparent that the parents had stuck to the decision not to respond to her phone calls more than one time each day. Monica had been very agitated by this decision and had reacted to the plan by crying and begging them to change it: "You don't understand; I *need* you to answer me; I can't help it." Their frustration stemmed from the fact that Monica continued to call each of them multiple times a day despite their determination not to answer. This seemed to mean that she was not able to handle the change and they were considering revising it.

In discussing the event with the parents they came to see that they and Monica had actually made tremendous progress. They had reflected to her an image of herself as a strong person capable of handling anxiety. And despite her calls, Monica had actually "survived" multiple days on which she did not talk to them repeatedly on the phone. The parents agreed that her mood did not seem more despondent and agreed to continue the process. The therapist asked the parents to count right then in the session the number of times Monica had called each of them each day. The parents pulled out their cell phones and were quite surprised to realize that the number had been dropping regularly.

Reinforcement for the Child

When reinforcements for the child have not been structured into the plan, the therapist should plan these in the first review session. Two main kinds of reinforcements are appropriate:

1. Reinforcement for positive behavior on the part of the child — for example, staying in their own bed, not asking questions, speaking to a stranger, and so on.
2. Reinforcement simply for having coped with changes the parents made. These are not contingent on the child *willingly* coping — they simply reflect the fact that they *have* coped.

Reinforcements can take many forms, including praise, prizes, shared activities, and others. Praise should be given generously and authentically — if the child spent one hour yelling, parents should probably not say, "You handled that with poise," but might say, "You got through it, and we're proud of you — it clearly was very hard." Even when a child has reacted in a negative or disruptive way to the parental steps, and there is a need to correct this behavior, the fact of having "gotten through it" remains unchanged.

> Bella was an 11-year-old girl who insisted on sleeping in her parents' bed and forbade them to turn off the light even after she was asleep. The parents informed her she was no longer allowed to sleep in their bed and that if she did they would leave her alone there. At night, Bella tried to lie down next to her mother and both parents reminded her of their decision. When she insisted, they left the room silently. Bella became very agitated and followed them around the house for more than an hour becoming increasingly abusive in her demands that they sleep next to her. Eventually, she became exhausted and fell asleep on the floor in her room. At breakfast she entered the kitchen with a sheepish look. Her mother hugged her and whispered in her ear "I'm proud of you." Bella looked confused, "I thought you would be mad at me for yesterday." Her mother responded, "It was wrong to talk to us like that but do you realize what you did last night? You slept all by yourself in your room! That's amazing! I'm just so proud."

When more material reinforcements are used, such as prizes or treats, these should be small enough to allow them to be repeated many times. Rather than promising a large prize for when a child becomes completely independent or makes very significant progress, parents should use very small reinforcements for every repetition of the desired coping behavior.

A Word on "Bribery"

A frequently voiced concern regarding the use of reinforcements, particularly tangible ones, is that this may represent a "bribe." What is meant by this is often not completely clear, but one worry is about creating an overly monetized relationship in which a child will only do things for prizes or will make ever increasing demands for reward. Although this is a valid concern, we advise parents to differentiate between two different kinds of reinforcement, which have been studied extensively in the field of behavior shaping.

One kind of reinforcement is given to a child as a means of stopping a negative and undesirable behavior. An example might be the child who is having a tantrum, which is distressing to the parents. In this case, by offering a child a reward in exchange for stopping the negative behavior the parents may unwittingly be actually reinforcing it. Children learn that by acting in that way they can earn a reward (for stopping), and the parents are actually being reinforced by the children for giving the reward (by gaining peace and quiet). This kind of reinforcement is clearly problematic and usually best avoided altogether.

A different kind of reward occurs when parents observe a positive behavior, which they hope to increase, and reinforce it by granting the child a reward. In this case it is the desired behavior that is most likely to be repeated. The possibility for overdependence on rewards does exist but can usually be mitigated. Most behavioral scientists agree that rewards are an effective way of shaping behavior and that long-term benefits outweigh the potential for negative outcomes.

Problem-Solve Difficulties

After reviewing the preceding week and reinforcing any progress, the therapist and the parents will identify key obstacles that were an impediment to implementing the parental plan. Ask parents to describe in detail the situations in which they felt least able to act as they meant to. Try to identify the facets of the situation most likely to have contributed to that feeling. These may include any number of variables such as being confused by the child's reaction, pressure to resolve a situation rapidly because of other obligations, or perhaps finding that they no longer think the plan was correctly formulated.

After identifying the factors contributing to the lack of success, attempt to problem-solve this event by considering the things that might have allowed it to have gone more smoothly. Would it have helped to disengage more successfully from argument? Would the presence of supporters in the home have made a difference? Should both parents have been more involved? Perhaps the plan should be modified to include a more gradual approach? Or conversely, perhaps parents should be making a "cleaner break" in their behavior? The goal of the therapist is to remain open to the possibility of a need to change the plan of action, but also able to withstand the frustration of difficult or uneven progress.

After problem-solving the situation, reformulate the plan and ensure that the revision is as specific as possible.

Plan for Next Steps

When parents have successfully implemented the plan to a substantial degree it will likely be appropriate to revise it for the coming week. This will reflect an additional step in the gradual process of reducing accommodation and promoting self-regulation and coping. Examples include increasing the length of time a parent leaves the child alone, further reducing parental participation in rituals, or reassurance or other increments and changes.

CONSIDER SESSION MODULES

- Recruiting and engaging supporters.
- Improving collaboration between parents.
- Dealing with extreme disruptive behavior.
- Dealing with threats of self-injury or suicide.
- Teaching the child anxiety regulation strategies.

PART VI: ADDITIONAL TARGETS—PARENTS TAKE THE LEAD

This session assumes that the parents have successfully modified their behavior with respect to the child's anxiety, leading to increased confidence and knowledge. When the parents have not yet successfully implemented changes, the therapy continues to follow Part III, implementing Session Modules as necessary. The goal of Part VI is to choose an additional target problem and to formulate a plan for addressing it. The parents are encouraged to take a more active role in preparing for informing the child (either in written or spoken form) and in formulating the plan to modify their accommodating behavior. This is particularly important as it will serve to build confidence in their ability to address additional challenges after the termination of parent guidance with the therapist.

Choosing a Target Problem

The same principles apply to choosing the second target problem as did in the first instance. Namely, the problem should be one that centers on parent accommodation, manifests frequently, poses significant interference to the function of child or family, and that parents are motivated to address. At this point parents may choose to ask children whether they feel there is an additional anxiety-related challenge that they would like to work on. Even children who were not amenable to collaborating on overcoming anxiety in earlier stages may be more receptive now. This can happen because the children have grown more confident of their own abilities or because they are more aware of their parents' determination and capability to further the process independently.

Informing the Child

Parents should discuss how best to inform the child of their intent to address the additional target problem (if the child has not been part of the decision process), and the therapist should guide the conversation, allowing them to build on the previous experience. Most commonly, the need for written communication will have decreased as parents and child have become accustomed to unilateral parental action. However, when communication is still strained or explosive reactions continue to be a factor, the written announcement should be used as described earlier. Parents should attempt to draft the announcement cooperatively, and the therapist should review and revise it with them.

Informing the child should always remain a reflection of the principles of the parental supportive stance:

- Acknowledgment of the child's fear and of the legitimacy of those feelings.
- Confidence in the child's ability to withstand anxiety.
- Description of the planned parental steps.
- Statement that these steps are not punitive but rather a means of helping the child and a reflection of their belief in the child's strength.

Dealing with Child Reactions

Parents and therapist discuss the possible reactions the child may exhibit to both the information and the actual steps and the ways in which these will be handled. Here, too, the therapist should be encouraging the parents to take a more active role in planning, basing their conversation on the content of earlier sessions. The main tools for overcoming child resistance will be:

Disengagement—A determination not to be drawn into argument, debate, or provocation. Parents should role-play, not answering the child when anxiety is causing him or her to draw them into unhelpful discussion.

Distancing—Parents should be prepared to distance themselves from situations of escalation, including explosive or disruptive behavior on the part of the child, physical or verbal aggression, or any behavior that will challenge their ability to preserve a determined equanimity.

Supporters—The involvement of additional figures in the process (as described in the relevant Session Module) can be a powerful tool for reducing escalation, facilitating communication, and preserving motivation.

Intersession Goals

1. Informing the child.
2. Implementing the plan formulated in the session.
3. Charting accommodation for the target problem. Parents should try to adhere successfully to the plan 100% of the time, but should

not be expected to be totally successful. They should monitor their successes and setbacks as well as the child's reactions.

CONSIDER SESSION MODULES

- Recruiting and engaging supporters.
- Improving collaboration between parents.
- Dealing with extreme disruptive behavior.
- Dealing with threats of self-injury or suicide.
- Teaching the child anxiety regulation strategies.

PART VII: ADDITIONAL TARGET—CONTINUED

This session reviews the parents' report of their progress regarding both target problems: the original problem and the newer one selected in the previous session.

Review of Informing the Child

For the newer target problem, parents first report on the child's reaction to their decision. Compare this reaction to the child's reaction the first time. What were the differences?

- Did the child seem more accepting?
- Did the child seem to have a greater awareness of the parents' motivation and determination?
- Did the parents feel differently this time? Were they more confident? Were they more or less hopeful than before?

Ask parents to reflect on these differences or similarities and to speculate on how they might feel in the future if they felt the need to address another related issue. What has the experience so far changed in their attitude toward themselves and their child?

Review of Parental Steps

For both target problems ask parents to review the situations they felt went the best, and those that posed the greatest challenges. Which target problem seemed the easier one for them to succeed with over the past week? Did adding an additional target make it more difficult to maintain the progress made so far?

Maintain a balance between discussion of positive and negative experiences. Avoid devoting all the time to discussing the times that were hardest or that went most easily. Maintaining balance allows for problem solving around difficult situations while preserving confidence and motivation.

Review of Child Reactions

For both target problems ask parents to describe the children's reactions to the modifications in their behavior. Did they note significant differences? If so, what do they think explains these differences?

Ask parents about any worrying or extreme reaction on the part of the child. Implement the relevant Session Modules on coping with extreme child behaviors if necessary.

Ask parents about any additional changes they have witnessed in the child that do not relate directly to the target problems. Have they noticed changes in mood? Increased or decreased flexibility in any areas of child functioning? New interests on the part of the child?

Reinforcing Progress

Discuss with the parents the progress that has been made over the past week as well as the overall progress over the course of treatment so far. The discussion should reflect the different kinds of progress that may have been made, and the therapist should be generous and genuine in praise for the parents.

Progress in Parents' Self-Efficacy

Parents may now be feeling more able to withstand the child's reactions or more able to help their child. This feeling of increased self-efficacy is an important change and should be stressed and reflected to them.

> You are taking a role of leadership and fulfilling an important parental role, I admire that.

By overcoming your fear, you are helping your child to overcome hers.

Progress in Reducing Accommodation and in Child's Coping

All too often parents and therapists alike tend to focus exclusively on what remains to be accomplished, while overlooking the changes already made. Recognizing the progress the parents have made constitutes a necessary reinforcement.

> Yes, he still has a ways to go, but you have shown the most important thing already: that he can get better, and that you can help him to do it.

Progress in Child's Ability to Withstand Anxiety

Reflect to the parents that positive changes in the child's reactions to their actions reflect increased tolerance for anxiety and better use of self-regulatory mechanisms.

> Teaching your child that they can cope with anxiety is giving them a wonderful gift, one they will need for the rest of their lives.

Progress in Overall Well-Being

Reflect to the parents any positive changes in the child that do not directly relate to the target problem but may result from better self-regulation or heightened self-esteem.

> It sounds like he is starting to see himself as more normal.

> You are helping her to feel better overall.

Reinforcement for the Child

Discuss the use of reinforcements for the child with regard to the new target problem. Allow parents to take the initiative in evaluating the possibilities in choosing reinforcements. The therapist should provide guidance to ensure that the principles of reinforcement described earlier are implemented. The reinforcements can include praise, shared activities, or tangible prizes. Actual prizes should be small and allow for consistent repetition. Parents should avoid using reinforcement as a means of stopping negative behaviors.

Plan for Next Steps

When parents have successfully implemented the plan to a substantial degree, it will likely be appropriate to revise it for the coming week. This will be reflected in additional steps in the gradual process of reducing accommodation and promoting self-regulation and coping. Examples include increasing the length of time a parent leaves the child alone, further reducing parental participation in rituals or reassurance or other increments and changes.

CONSIDER SESSION MODULES

- Recruiting and engaging supporters.
- Improving collaboration between parents.
- Dealing with extreme disruptive behavior.
- Dealing with threats of self-injury or suicide.
- Teaching the child anxiety regulation strategies.

PART VIII: SUMMARY AND TERMINATION

The Goals of the Final Part

1. Review the changes in child's anxiety symptoms—including targeted and nontargeted behaviors.
2. Review changes in parental attitudes and skills learned by parents.
3. Discuss additional goals parents would like to achieve.
4. Discuss maintaining progress and dealing with future exacerbations.

Review the Changes in Child's Anxiety Symptoms—Including Targeted and Nontargeted Behaviors

Ask parents to describe the changes they see in their child's anxiety-related symptoms, relative to before treatment:

How much has changed?

What has not improved?

Is the child better able to cope with the situations that triggered the parents' participation in treatment?

Are there additional domains of functioning that have improved?

Does the child seem more or less confident and competent overall?

Use the accommodation chart and refer back to the first accommodation chart completed by parents in Part III. How similar or different are the changes for each parent? Are there differences in sibling accommodation?

Review Changes in Parental Attitudes and Skills Learned by Parents

Ask parents to describe how they think about anxiety today and whether that has changed since starting treatment:

Do they think of their child as more capable of coping with anxiety?

Do they think differently now about their own roles as parents?

What would they say to the parents of another child who is overly anxious—has that changed?

Are they more in agreement between themselves about how to deal with their child's anxiety?

Do they feel better prepared to deal with anxiety in the future?

Are they less anxious themselves?

Ask parents to describe the main skills they can take away with them from treatment. Do they think they have more tools for handling anxiety? Remind parents of skills utilized in treatment:

- Decreasing argument and the use of written communication.
- Ability to make changes without child approval.
- Formulating and implementing a practical behavioral plan.
- Use of supporters.
- Dealing with disruptive or self-injurious behaviors or threats.
- Disengagement.
- Sit-in.

Ask parents if they feel they would be able to use the same skills without your supervision? Which ones? Are there skills they do not feel they understood or are not able to implement?

Discuss Additional Goals Parents Would Like to Achieve
Ask parents what anxiety-related symptoms they still feel need to be worked on and addressed at this point. It is normal for there to be additional symptoms (child avoidance, family accommodation, dysregulation) that remain after treatment.

Remind parents that anxiety is normal and the goal is not to have a child "without anxiety," but a child who is better able to cope with anxiety. Emphasize that this will better prepare the child for dealing with challenges in the future.

Ask parents if they feel competent to tackle these remaining symptoms outside of the context of parent guidance sessions. Ask them to describe how they think they will do that.

Discuss the potential for individual treatment with the child at this point, or in the future. Has the child expressed an interest in participating in treatment? A common outcome of good parent work is the child's growing motivation for treatment. Explain that this demonstrates both an increased sense of hope that she can overcome problems if she gets help, and a greater acceptance of the idea that avoidance and accommodation are not an option. Help parents to plan for treatment if warranted.

Discuss Maintaining Progress and Dealing with Future Exacerbations
Maintaining Gains Explain to parents that there is a likelihood that the child will resume some of the avoidance that has been diminished, if the opportunity exists. For example, a child who has become able to sleep alone might ask to sleep in the parents' bed again. A child who has returned to school might ask to stay home for one day. Encourage parents not to confuse the child by accommodating behaviors they have struggled to change.

Your child will still feel anxious some of the time, and may try to "test the waters" to see if he or she can resume some of the previous behavioral patterns. This does not reflect something bad and almost all children will

205

be compelled to make at least one such attempt. You can show them that you still believe in them and are confident they can handle the anxiety.

Do not be afraid to rock the boat! In other words, do not try to keep things going smoothly by allowing the child to relapse. If you are confident and determined, the challenge will pass much more quickly than if you confuse the child by making changes and going backward. You might say in a supportive way, "We see you are feeling a little anxious about that again. That's normal but we know you can handle this."

Future Exacerbations Explain that a child who has a tendency to be overly anxious is likely to encounter that tendency again in the future. This might happen soon, or it could occur farther down the road. It also might not happen at all but it is reasonable to expect that the child will have to overcome anxiety again. Emphasize that by overcoming the current problem, parents have taught themselves and the child a valuable lesson: They can get over the anxiety!

Discuss what steps the parents will take if they recognize signs of elevated anxiety in the future. These might include:

- Implementing the tools learned in the SPACE Program.
- Contacting the therapist.
- Resuming parent guidance.
- Treatment for the child.

CHAPTER TWELVE

Tools for Troubleshooting the SPACE Program

Session Modules

Working with parents can present a variety of challenges for which the therapist must be prepared. This chapter includes Session Modules—strategies for troubleshooting some common obstacles to treating childhood anxiety through parent work with the SPACE Program.

Key points in this chapter:

- Teaching the child regulation strategies.
- Improving collaboration between parents.
- Recruiting and engaging supporters.
- Dealing with extreme disruptive behavior.
- Dealing with threats of self-injury or suicide.

SESSION MODULE—TEACHING THE CHILD ANXIETY REGULATION STRATEGIES

The goal of this module (which may be presented in parts rather than as a whole) is to teach parents anxiety regulation strategies, which they can teach the child, if the child is responsive and collaborative. The anxiety regulation strategies include tools that target the emotional, cognitive, and physiological aspects of anxiety.

Explain to parents that the tools should be taught to children to help them cope with anxiety caused by their decreased accommodation, as well as for them to use whenever feeling anxious. Explain also to the parents that the tools can help them deal with their own anxiety and help them gain better control over their own reactions.

Explain that every child is different and the best strategy for one child may not work well for another, or may simply seem less interesting or attractive to a specific child. Encourage them to propose the strategies in an open, noncoercive way, allowing children to explore and express what works best for them.

Relaxing Breathing

Explain to parents that by relaxing the body children can regulate anxiety, causing them to feel less afraid and to think less anxious thoughts. Relaxing breathing can be a powerful tool. Explain that when children are anxious their breathing will be affected, and by reversing those changes anxiety is reduced. Children often need to practice relaxation a number of times when they are not particularly stressed, before being able to implement the technique at times of heightened anxiety. Once the skill has been mastered and they are more competent at regulating their internal physiological level of arousal, children will be able to use the skill either as a regular part of their routine, increasing overall well-being, or as a more "S.O.S" kind of tool—to be used when they feel afraid.

The main goal in relaxing breathing (also called *diaphragmatic breathing* or *abdominal breathing*) is to breathe in such a way that the abdomen, rather than the chest, expands to make room for the increased volume of the lungs. This is counterintuitive for many children who are used to pulling their shoulders back and puffing out their chest to take a deep breath. In fact, many children will actually suck their belly in while inhaling—the opposite of the desired effect. Placing a hand on one's abdomen while doing the exercise or lying down with a small soft toy on the belly can provide cues to whether the abdomen is moving in the right direction.

Ask the parents to practice relaxing breathing with you to learn the technique and be able to teach it to the child. The following text can be used to instruct the parents on relaxing breathing and they can use the same text when teaching the child:

> First we're going to breathe out all the air in our lungs. Let the air out slowly through your mouth. Breathe it out slowly as though you were using a soap bubble toy and wanted to make a really big bubble without letting it pop. As we breathe out we are going to push our belly in, toward the back, with our hand. Not too hard, just squeezing it back a little. When we feel like we need to breathe in again we'll take in air through our nose. As we do, we'll let our belly rise back up again as though being puffed up with the air we're breathing in. Let's do it together. Slowly breathe out and push your belly back. Wait a few seconds. . . . Now breathe in and let your belly puff out again.

Cognitive Restructuring

Explain to parents that cognitive restructuring refers to the practice of identifying the anxious thoughts that are making a child fearful and then challenging those thoughts with more realistic estimations and assessments. Parents can teach the child to engage in cognitive restructuring and then practice with the child when anxious thoughts occur or as preparation for a situation that is likely to trigger them.

First practice with the parents and then they will be able to re-create the experience with the child. Have the parents say some of the thoughts that make their child anxious. For example, a parent might say, "Whenever he or someone in the family gets sick, he thinks it will be a serious disease and that they might die." Have the parents challenge the anxious thoughts by formulating questions that target their accuracy or likelihood. Write down the anxious thought on one side of a paper. For example, they might write: "If someone is sick it is very serious and they will die." Have the parent write down on the other side of the paper the challenging questions and a more reasonable thought, not one that is overly optimistic (e.g., "No one in my family will get seriously ill"), but one that is more realistic. For example, they might write: "Most of the time people get better pretty soon," or "I've been sick lots of times and it wasn't a big deal in the end."

Most parents are already engaging in this kind of dialogue with their children as a means of reassuring them, but cognitive restructuring is not about their *telling* them a reassuring thought, but about the children juxtaposing their own anxious ideation with more realistic cognitions and practicing doing it repeatedly when anxious thoughts appear. Below are some other examples of cognitive restructuring.

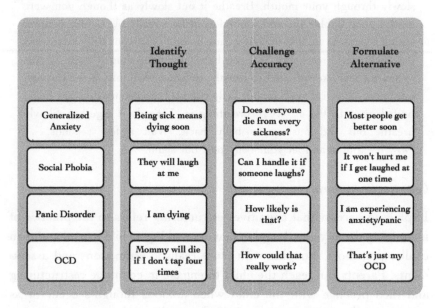

Examples of cognitive restructuring illustrating the strategy for various anxiety disorders.

Guided Imagery

Explain to parents that children who are anxious are being tormented by their imagination. Their imagination produces thoughts, pictures, and scenarios of negative events, and they feel anxious or avoid the situation in which those things might happen. But the imagination can be a tool the child can use to actually feel *less* anxious. One way in which children can use their imagination is by visualizing how the disturbing thought wanes, gets smaller and smaller, and eventually vanishes. As children watch their thoughts growing farther and farther away the effect can be a dramatic reduction in anxiety.

The following script is one example of using the imagination to reduce anxiety in this way. Practice this with the parents in the session using a thought that would be anxiety-provoking to them. Ask them to first try to make themselves a little anxious by focusing on the negative thoughts. Help the parents to experience some elevated anxiety by discussing their fear a little. Then ask them to assume a relaxed and comfortable position in their chair and slowly present the following imagery:

> Imagine a field—a green, wide field stretched as far as you can see. And over the field the sky is blue and clear like on a really nice day. Try to see the colors of the field and the sky. Feel the light breeze in the air and try to smell the scent of the fresh ground and clean air. Now imagine a hot air balloon floating over this field, gently drifting across the sky from directly above you and moving across the field, heading off toward the horizon. In the basket hanging from under the balloon I want you to place the thought that is troubling you right now. You can put it there any way you like. You could imagine writing it on paper and placing that there, or imagine a picture of your thought in the basket or just imagine that you have placed your thought there in some way. Now watch as the balloon drifts gently away from you, going farther and farther and taking your thought with it. Soon you can hardly see the balloon or the thought at all and then it disappears entirely. Now, if you like you can summon another balloon and put another thought on it. Watch as it too drifts slowly away over the field. You can put as many thoughts as you like or you can put the same thought in again if it still is bothering you and watch until it disappears again.

Harness Feelings

Explain to the parents that feelings and emotions don't have to be controlled by the anxiety; they can be controlled by the child. They can actually be tools for children to make themselves feel less anxious. It is difficult for children to feel at once very scared and also very angry, so the parents can teach children to start getting mad at the fear—and then they'll feel less afraid.

Ask the parents to help their children make a sock puppet that will represent anxiety. They can give it a funny name, draw a face on it, or use their creativity in any other way. The parents will explain to children that when anxiety starts making them feel bad they can take the anxiety-puppet and "teach it a lesson." Ask the parents to encourage children to be as expressive as possible about their anger at the puppet. They could yell at it; scream as loud as they can; throw it down on the floor and stomp up and down on it; punch it as hard as they can; or squeeze it until it's totally crushed. Explain to the parents that directing anger at the puppet in this way is positive and not misbehavior. The angrier children get at the fear, the less afraid they will feel—and the more motivated not to give in to it.

Session Module—Improving Collaboration Between Parents

This Session Module is meant to be included in the course of the SPACE Program when parents have difficulty working collaboratively together. Therapists should be aware of the strain that a child's anxiety disorder can place on the marital relationship as well as of the impact that a lack of cooperation can have on the course of treatment. However, the treatment overall must remain focused on addressing the anxiety and not take on a primary role of couples counseling.

The goals of this session are to:

- Identify the main sources of discord between parents in addressing the child's anxiety.
- Suggest means of improving collaboration.

Identify Sources of Discord

When disagreement between parents is evident in the parent guidance process, the therapist should aim to first identify some of the main factors contributing to the discord. These can include many different factors, such as different opinions about what constitutes healthy or acceptable functioning, different ideas about how to respond to anxiety, divergent parenting styles, or unrelated marital stressors that are impacting overall collaboration.

Ask the parents how they feel the other spouse is acting with regard to the anxiety, and whether they would change that behavior if they could. Ask parents whether they feel that their partner is supportive of their efforts or possibly undermines them, with regard to the anxiety. Inquire

212

about the amounts of time each parent spends with the child and about the kind of time (i.e., entertainment, chores, homework, or bedtime). Differential exposure to the anxiety or the need of one parent to confront it more often, can lead to a lack of harmony and to feelings of resentment.

Many couples experience tension because one parent is attempting to demand more independent functioning from the child and feels that the other is being overly protective or is "giving in to the anxiety." In that case the more demanding parents may believe that their spouse is being manipulated by the child, who is using anxiety as a means of imposing demands or merely seeking attention. The other, less demanding, parents may feel that only they are providing the child with a sense of reassurance or are acknowledging what the child is feeling.

Strategies for Increasing Collaboration

Below are a number of strategies for improving parents' ability to work together collaboratively. The goal is not to create perfect harmony or to ensure that both parents agree about all the issues. Rather the therapist aims to reduce conflict and to create a collaborative environment in which both parents can recognize the value of cooperation while maintaining their individual points of view.

Integrate Parental Stances—Remember That Support Includes Both
Acknowledgment and Confidence
When the two parents are divided, as is often the case, by one being more reassuring and empathic and the other being more demanding of the child's coping, it is easy for parents to see themselves as working for the better and the others as "damaging" the situation. However, the SPACE Program defines support of an anxious child as the successful integration of *both* those two elements. Only when parents are combining acceptance and acknowledgment of the child's fear and distress with a belief in the child's ability to withstand gradually greater degrees of anxiety, are they conveying support. Therefore, while each parent may feel the other is missing the point, in fact both are bringing to the situation a vital element of support.

By helping parents to recognize this, the degree of antagonism between parents can be minimized and more productive cooperation can be fostered. Rather than parents each seeing the other as hurting the child and undermining themselves, they can appreciate the value of the added element and attempt to integrate it with those ideas that are more intuitively accessible to them. Integrating the parental stances in this way will promote the efficacy of the more practical tools described below.

Plan in Session—Implement at Home

When parents are having trouble communicating or working cooperatively, the need to plan their actions together with the therapist during the session, rather than relying on more flexible or spontaneous decision making at home, becomes imperative. During the SPACE Program sessions, parents work to come up with a plan with which they both identify and that feels comfortable to both, so as to minimize the need for cooperative decision making at home. No plan can foresee every eventuality, but the more specific the planning during the sessions the less opportunity and need the parents will have to improvise at home.

The therapist should be careful to ensure that both parents actually do agree with the plan formulated during the session. In one case a therapist worked with the parents to operationalize their decreased accommodation and was not aware that actually only the father was taking an active role, while the mother was mostly silent. The next week the father complained that his spouse had not worked as agreed. The mother responded, "This was never my plan to begin with! The two of you decided it without my consent." By consistently engaging both parents in the process, the therapist can lower the likelihood of similar events occurring in the treatment.

Setting Aside a Time for Communication

The therapist should work with the parents to plan a specific time (daily or a few times a week) during which to communicate information and feelings about the progress they are making. As is the case in many areas of discontent, parents are most likely to bring up their frustration when it is actually being triggered. For example, a mother who feels her spouse is being overly demanding or critical of her, may say this when faced with an instance of harsh criticism. Unfortunately, it is exactly at these moments that communication is actually least likely to be helpful, and that escalation in the conversation between the parents is most predictably going to occur. This has the effect of turning the conversation into an argument, in which both sides feel attacked or disappointed. After this fruitless conversation, many parents will then ignore the problem until the next time the emotions are powerfully triggered. This pattern ensures that the cooperation continues to deteriorate and that progress will be severely hampered.

By setting aside a specific time, during which parents will share information and impressions about the child's coping, discuss how they are handling the implementation of the plan, and even voice opinions about how the other spouse is doing, the likelihood of breakdown is mitigated.

Role Play—Switching Places

This is an exercise designed to help parents appreciate the value of the other parent's point of view, and reduce antagonism in the relationship. The point of the exercise is for each parent to adopt the role of the other— for a set amount of time. For example, when a mother has been focusing on reassuring and comforting her child when she is upset, and the father has been directing his efforts toward teaching the daughter that she can cope with her fear and need not seek the parents' protection—the roles can be temporarily reversed. Here is an example of a text the therapist can use to instruct the parents in the role play (used with the parents of an 8-year-old boy who spent every night in his parents' bed):

> For one night I would like to ask you to "change places," to switch roles. You, mom, have been working so hard to make sure that Kyle feels comforted at night and that he can rely on you. You will be responsible— for just this one night—for helping Kyle to see that he can handle being anxious even if he doesn't sleep next to you. Remember this is only for just the one night. You, dad, have been trying hard to make sure Kyle overcomes his fear and does not rely too much on your presence or reassurance. Just for tonight, you will have another job—you will simply try to help him to feel loved, accepted, and comforted. For this one night you will not try to make him better, only make him feel better.

Parents who engage in this kind of exercise often feel a greater appreciation of the goal the other parent is trying to achieve. Many parents recognize that, in fact, they too share their spouse's goal, but have been completely focused on what they see as a more pressing and incompatible objective. The idea of support demonstrates that the two goals are in fact compatible, and the exercise allows the parents to reconnect with both elements.

Session Module—Recruiting and Engaging Supporters

This Session Module will be a part of almost all SPACE Program implementations and is modular because its location in the sequence of sessions can vary. The default location will be as a fourth or fifth session, but in some cases it may be introduced earlier or later in the process. When a family is faced with, or foresees, particularly disruptive reactions on the part of the child or threats of self-injury or suicide, the presence of supporters is integral to dealing with these problems. In other cases the use of supporters will be primarily as a means of advancing the treatment process.

The goals of the session are to:

- Introduce the concept of supporters and the rationale for their use.
- Introduce the roles supporters can fulfill.
- Create a list of potential supporters (can also be an intersession goal).
- Instruct parents on recruiting supporters and explaining their role to them.

Introducing the Concept of Supporters

The support of people outside of the child's immediate nuclear family can be a powerful tool in promoting progress and overcoming obstacles. The therapist should introduce the five following potentially helpful roles that supporters can fill:

1. Supporters can help to reinforce the parental message regarding the need to overcome the anxiety. Children may see the parents' efforts as either an attack against them or as idiosyncratic to those

216

parents—something others would not agree with. When a significant number of other individuals convey to the child that what the parents are doing is necessary and merely reflects their responsibility as parents, these views are less likely to be maintained.

2. By expressing caring and concern for children, and confidence in their abilities, supporters can bolster the children's self-esteem and encourage motivation.

3. Supporters can help children in confronting situations they fear. Although children look to their parents for protection and reassurance, they are often actually more fearful in their parents' presence. This is because they are using the parent as a regulator of their inner state rather than attempting to overcome the obstacle themselves. In the presence of supporters other than the parents, children may be more willing to face a frightening situation.

4. Supporters can help to mediate between parents and child and can promote the child's collaboration with the process. Although emotional tension can run high between parents and children, leading to breakdowns in communication, others may be more able to maintain a productive dialogue.

5. Supporters can help to minimize disruptive behavior and to react to such behaviors in effective ways that do not escalate the situation. This is discussed more fully in the *Session Module on dealing with extreme disruptive behavior.*

For some parents, the involvement of supporters from outside the home can be a difficult decision and the therapist's suggestions may be met with initial resistance. Empathy for the parents' concerns will allow them to discuss their apprehension and work through it together with the therapist. Most commonly, parents resist involving supporters for some of the following reasons.

Fear of Violating the Privacy of the Child or the Family
Although a right to growing degrees of privacy is part of normal development, it is helpful to remind parents that this should not override the child's even more basic right to parents' commitment to help in overcome challenges and difficulties. Remind the parents that the goal of the supporters is not to shame children or embarrass them but rather to

rally round the children, giving them the message: "We all care about you, believe in you, and are going to help you."

Fear of Criticism by the Supporters
This fear is almost always greatly overestimated. When asked for help, the majority of individuals invariably focus less on castigating the parents for prior mistakes and more on helping them to overcome the problem. In fact, many supporters openly express admiration for the parents' decision not to ignore the problem and not to let their own embarrassment stand in the way of helping the child. Many supporters will also, when approached, share similar difficulties they faced with their own children.

Fear of a Sense of Parental Failure
It is a fallacy of modern parenting that problems should be resolved in the confines of the immediate nuclear family, and that any difficulty in doing so indicates a shortcoming on the part of the parents. In fact, as expressed by the proverb made famous by Hillary Clinton "It takes a village to raise a child," there is always a need for support from the community. The belief that benefiting from help and support are equivalent to failure cuts both parent and child off from what can be tremendously helpful resources.

Fear of the Child's Reaction
For many parents the main source of apprehension is the fear that involving supporters will trigger negative reactions on the part of the child. These may include outbursts of anger and rage, exacerbations in the child's symptoms or potential harm to the child's existing relationship with the supporters. Experience has shown that these fears are greatly exaggerated. As in most other cases, refraining from doing the necessary thing because of a fear of recrimination only serves to worsen the problem at hand. In this case, children learn that by threatening negative outcomes they can ensure that their parents will not pursue their intentions. This is not only a negative message but also leaves children knowing that they have little hope of getting better. With regard to children's relationships with the supporters, there can in fact be temporary deleterious effects, as when children decide they do not want to speak with that person

218

anymore or feel embarrassed that they know about the disorder. Nevertheless, in the longer run the relationship is generally strengthened when the supporters show their dedication to helping the child and a lack of judgment of the anxiety.

Creating a List of Potential Supporters

Work with the parents to come up with a list of as many people as possible who can take on the role of supporters. Typically, the list will include relatives such as uncles, aunts, and grandparents; friends of the family who have known the child for some time; individuals such as sports coaches and guidance counselors; primary care providers and others.

Reassure the parents that, although some of the supporters may take on active roles, this is not a necessity and most will likely only have to provide minimal effort to actually be helpful. Supporters do not have to be individuals with any special psychological training or insight and they do not need to command the child's respect and obedience. They merely will have to be willing to take some part in the process, and therapists, directly or indirectly, will provide practical information on how to implement their involvement. Supporters also do not all have to live in the vicinity of the family. In fact, some can actually be located in remote locations such as other countries. The therapist should encourage the parents to include, however, at least some supporters who do live close to them.

In most cases the list will include between 5 and 10 supporters and there is no maximum number of supporters. Having less than five altogether would be less desirable.

Recruiting the Supporters

The therapist should encourage the parents to contact the entire list of supporters and to explain to them the reason for the request. Parents should be open about the fears children have been experiencing and the impact that they have had on them and on the family. They should state that as part of their effort to help children overcome these fears they are participating in a program of parent guidance, and that their therapist has recommended that they try to engage the help of some individuals who may be willing to lend a hand. The parents should make clear that the role of supporter will not entail great effort and will not interfere with any of their regular commitments or activities.

Supporters' Roles

The open and consistent use of supporters can greatly facilitate the successful implementation of the SPACE Program. Here are some of the ways in which supporters can be utilized over the course of treatment.

Expressing Support

The first role that supporters will usually fill is to contact the child and let him or her know that they are aware of the problem. Supporters should clearly state that the child is important to them, that they care about him or her, and that they understand his or her fear and suffering. However, the supporter should also explicitly state that the child's parents must act to solve the problem, and that is why they turned to them. If supporters do not feel comfortable going to the child personally, or if they are separated by distance, this can be done by phone, letter, fax, text, or by email. In this manner they can give significant support even if they are in another country.

Offering Help

If supporters have a positive relationship with the child, they can offer to talk to him or her about the anxiety or to help in any other way the child wishes. This can be important in defining the supporters as providing support *for the child* rather than only for the parents, and can help a child to feel more hopeful and less alone.

Intervening in Crisis

See the Session Module on dealing with extreme disruptive behavior.

Reinforcing Progress

Supporters can reinforce children's progress when this occurs by calling to praise them, giving them a reward, or spending fun time with them during which time they can also discuss the progress.

Support for Parents

Parents will face difficult moments, during which they will need to overcome the urge to accommodate the child because of distress, time constraints, or exhaustion. Supporters can be available to the parents in these moments by phone or in person to offer encouragement and support. Sometimes, saying something as simple as, "Let's meet right now and have a coffee," or "This is a really tough time, tomorrow you'll be proud of yourself for persevering," will be sufficient to help a parent through a stressful moment.

SESSION MODULE—DEALING WITH EXTREME DISRUPTIVE BEHAVIOR

This Session Module is meant to be included in the SPACE Program when a child exhibits overly aggressive or disruptive behavior, in response to the parents' plans or actions. When prior experience indicates that such behavior is likely, it should be included as part of the preparation process (along with *formulating a plan*), and introducing this module should precede any actual steps taken by the parents, including the announcement. This Session Module assumes the presence and engagement of supporters, and should always be preceded by the Session Module *Recruiting and Utilizing Supporters*.

The goal of the session is to prepare parents to respond to disruptive behavior in a way that reduces the likelihood of its recurrence and does not escalate the behavior in the short term. The session includes:

- Describing the behavior.
- Introducing the concept of delayed response.
- The sit-in.
- Supporters in the context of disruptive behaviors.

Describing the Disruptive Behavior

Ask parents to describe the disruptive behavior that has occurred in response to their actions, or that they fear will occur. Help parents to be as specific as possible and reduce embarrassment or discomfort by normalizing the presence of disruptive behavior. Violent or aggressive behavior should be framed as an expression of anxiety, rather than as indicative of an inherently belligerent personality, whenever appropriate. State specifically that a child acting in a disruptive way is not a sign of failed parenting or of a flawed personality.

221

We need to remember that the anxiety response is one of "fight or flight"—that includes fight! Lots of people react aggressively when they're anxious.

When she is less anxious it is likely that her aggressive behavior will also get much better. We need to make sure that the aggressive behavior itself doesn't stop that from happening.

The description of the behavior should include:

The Kinds of Behaviors Displayed

Is the child physically violent?
In what ways is he violent?
Is he verbally abusive?
Who are the targets of the behavior (parents, siblings, others)?
Is he violent toward property?

The Triggers

What provokes the disruptive behavior?
Does she respond violently to certain statements?
Do certain situations make the violence much more likely?

The Setting

Where does the disruptive behavior occur?
Is it most likely to happen at home?
Does it happen in other locations?

Prior Parental Responses

What steps have you taken in the past to respond to the disruptive behavior?
Have those responses been effective at stopping the behavior?
Have they prevented it from recurring again in the future?

Introduce the Concept of Delayed Response

Explain that most reactions to a child's disruptive behavior, that occur while the child is being disruptive, tend to backfire. In other words, they make things worse (more disruptive behavior) rather than better (less disruptive behavior). Explain to the parents that there are several reasons for why immediate responses often backfire and review with them those that follow.

Child Is in a State of Heightened Arousal
When children are acting in aggressive or disruptive ways they are experiencing heightened, at times extreme, emotional and physical arousal that significantly alters their perception and interpretation of events. When feeling combative, even relatively innocuous cues, such as a parent saying "You need to calm down now," may seem to the child to represent a threat or a challenge. Cognitive processing is impaired in this condition, as is the ability to accurately discern the intentions of others (a process termed *mentalization*).

Parent Is Under Stress
Children are not the only ones experiencing arousal when they are acting in a disruptive fashion. The stress of the situation, often exacerbated by a sense of failure, embarrassment, or frustration, will also have an effect on the parent. Parents, under these conditions, are more likely to act in impulsive or exaggerated ways, which tend to lead to escalation.

There Really Are No "Good Responses"
The feeling that a successful and effective parent would respond to aggression in "the perfect way" is no more than an illusion. In fact, this is part of a greater illusion that parents have the capacity, and by consequence the responsibility, to directly control a child's behavior. The truth, however, is that even the best parent cannot directly control the behavior of children, including making them stop acting out. By accepting this fact, parents are relieved of an impossible chore and free to choose more productive ways to respond.

The concept of **delayed response** reflects an acceptance of these limitations. Parents are not expected to be able to manage the disruptive situation, and instead focus on *getting through it*. Their only role while the child is acting in the disruptive manner is to ensure physical safety and resist being drawn into the interaction. If children voice a threat to the parents, they should avoid responding in kind (i.e., "You'll be sorry if you do . . ."). Instead they should remain silent, or merely state in a quiet way that the behavior is unacceptable. If necessary, parents should attempt to distance themselves from the child in order to minimize the potential for escalation.

Parents may feel concerned that their refusal to respond to the child's provocation represents an abdication of their parental role. The therapist can reassure the parents that they are not refusing to respond. They are merely refusing to become drawn into a hopeless situation. In fact, the most important response the parents can make is simply continuing the process of fostering better coping and self-regulation in the child. By seeing the explosive behavior as a child's way of saying "You see, you are making a mistake! You should not go ahead with this!" it becomes clear that the parent's determination to continue helping the child is the most effective response of all.

The Sit-In: Delayed Response to Disruptive Behavior

The sit-in is an act performed by parents in response to particularly disruptive behavior. It is performed in a way that conveys opposition to the behavior and commitment to eliminating it, without escalating the conflict between parents and child. The sit-in should only be performed in response to severe behaviors such as physical violence. Other, more minor negative behaviors, which result from parents pursuing the SPACE Program, should be ignored or responded to in the way parents normally do.

Explain to parents that the sit-in should not be performed immediately following the negative behavior, or while it is occurring, but rather at least a few hours later. It can even be performed the next day. This will also allow parents to better prepare for the sit-in, and for both parents to be present.

During the sit-in, both parents enter the child's room calmly, sit down, state the reason for their presence, and remain silently in the room for a significant amount of time (between half an hour and one hour). They do not engage in conversation but will leave the room if the child offers a solution to the problem of the negative behavior.

Explaining the Sit-In to Parents

Prepare for the sit-in by finding a time when both of you can be available, and free of other occupations, for 1 hour. If necessary, ask someone else or a babysitter to be in the home to look after siblings. Do not start the sit-in when you are feeling very angry about the behavior. Wait until you have calmed down. This will also help to make sure your child is less upset, too.

Enter the child's room and sit down. In a soft voice, state that you are there because of the child's behavior and that you are determined to solve this problem. Be specific about the behavior that has caused you to come. For example:

"Yesterday, when we did not agree to tell your friends you were not home, you acted violently. You hit your mother and broke her iPad. This is unacceptable and we will stay here now and wait for you to suggest a solution to this problem. We are not punishing you, but we cannot accept violence in our home."

Remain silently in the child's room for the rest of the duration of the sit-in. Do not ask him any more questions, and do not respond to arguments or provocation. If the child asks or tells you to leave, simply remain seated quietly.

If your child offers what seems like a reasonable solution, stand up, say, "Okay, we are going to try that" and leave the room. Do not talk about the sit-in after it is over. Even if the child retracts his solution after the sit-in, do not respond unless the behavior itself is repeated. In that case perform another sit-in but do not leave if the same solution is suggested again.

Duration: The sit-in should be adapted to the age of the child. For children under age 8, 20 minutes are sufficient; for children ages 8 to 12, half an hour; for children over age 13, 1 hour.

Supporters in the Context of Disruptive Behaviors

The recruitment of supporters, along with additional roles they can fulfill, is described in Session Module *Recruiting and Engaging Supporters*.

Disclosure Instead of Secrecy

Ask the parents to contact the supporters after each occurrence of aggressive or violent behavior and to inform them in detail of the event. Email can be used as a means of facilitating this process, by creating a group email that is sent after each event.

The child should be made explicitly aware of the fact that parents are sharing the details of the behavior with the supporters. If email is used the child should be copied on the email or a copy can be printed and given to him. If other means are used, the parents should create a log of the violent or aggressive behavior and present the child with a copy, including a list of the supporters who received the same information.

Any objection on the part of the child to this step should be met with a simple statement: "When you act in a violent way, we will not keep that a secret." Parents should adamantly avoid any further discussion of this point.

Supporters Contact the Child and Address the Behavior
Supporters should make contact with the child and express the following things:

- Their positive regard of the child.
- Their knowledge of the aggressive behavior—this should include specifics of the behavior.
- Their view that this behavior is unacceptable and support for parental steps.
- An offer to help the child.

Sample Text for Supporter   Fiona, I really like you and think you're a great kid. I heard from your mom and dad that you acted violently the other day. You hit them and used words like "asshole." I want you to know that even if you were feeling bad that kind of behavior is not something that's ever okay. I know your parents are trying to help you get better at handling things and I really support them. I also would really like to help you if I can. If there is any way I might help at all please let me know.

Sample Text for Supporter II   In another example a neighbor might address a child as follows:

> Gary, I know you are a good boy. The past few nights I have heard from my house the way you have been acting. I even saw you run into the street after your parents. I know you must have been really upset but that

kind of behavior is not good. It is dangerous. I think your parents are doing their job, trying to help you, but if I can help in some way I would love to try. Perhaps there is something you'd like me to tell them?

Supporters can use any means to contact the child, such as coming to the house for a visit or calling on the phone. Many children will naturally avoid talking with someone about their inappropriate behavior and contact can become more difficult after the first time. Supporters can choose to text, send an email or a letter, or even stand outside the child's room and simply state their message from behind a closed door. The important thing is that the child knows that they are aware of the problem, support the parents, and wish to help.

Supporters Can Help to Prevent Escalation

When triggers have been identified that predict the outburst of disruptive behaviors (such as the parental refusal to accommodate), supporters can be used to minimize the probability of escalation. The mere presence of supporters in the home when the situation arises will usually prevent the most problematic behaviors.

Parents can either simply have the supporters present or state their purpose explicitly to the child. For example, parents might say: "We asked your uncle to be here because we realized you might feel so bad you would react in an inappropriate way."

The role of supporters *is not* to actively prevent the violence. They should not intervene physically (apart from immediate danger) and should not lecture the child, but rather simply be present in a nonconfrontational manner. If challenged by the child they can state quietly, "I am only here to observe because your parents feared the situation might get out of hand." If the child continues to challenge them, they should avoid engaging in debate.

Supporters Can Facilitate Communication

Another role in which supporters can be helpful is as mediators, facilitating communication between parents and child. Children who refuse to collaborate directly with their parents and respond aggressively to unilateral action may be more amenable to discussion with a different person. Once children have accepted that the parents are determined to proceed despite their opposition, they may use the supporters as a way of climbing down from the tree of total resistance. Agreeing to collaborate through the supporters can be experienced as less of a "surrender" than directly conceding to work with the parents. This is particularly true of adolescent children.

SESSION MODULE—DEALING WITH THREATS OF SELF-INJURY OR SUICIDE

This Session Module is meant to be included in the SPACE Program when a child reacts to the parents' actions with threats of suicide or self-injury. When actual suicidal or self-injurious behavior has been previously exhibited, implementation of the SPACE Program should not be undertaken without close collaboration with psychiatric care. This Session Module may be incorporated into another session or may take up an entire session itself, depending on the level of threat and the amount of time necessary to adequately prepare the parents for dealing with it.

Creating a Supportive Parental Stance Regarding Threats to Self

Many parents, when faced with threats on the part of the child toward himself, will respond in one of two ways, both of which are unlikely to be helpful in resolving the situation.

Anxious Paralysis

This describes the parent who is overcome with feelings of fear of what the child may do, or of guilt at having triggered the threat. The feelings may be so powerful that the parent feels unable to take any real action and retreats into passivity. This kind of reaction, while lowering the child's immediate level of distress, does not improve the longer-term outcomes. Parents are likely to be perceived by children as unable to manage their emotion, and children learn that the threats, whether genuinely intended or not, are an effective way of dissuading the parents from determined action.

Confrontational Challenging

This describes the parent who feels convinced the child is "bluffing" and is compelled to "call the bluff." For example, when a child threatened to kill himself in response to one parent's actions, the parent responded by saying, "There's the window, you can jump anytime." This kind of response poses a dangerous taunt to children, who may feel humiliated or experience a loss of face if they do not accept the dare. Even children who were not at great risk for self-harm may feel trapped into behaviors they would not otherwise have performed.

What both of these responses have in common, despite being different, is that they do not face the new challenge in a supportive way. As described throughout this treatment, support is equal to combining an acknowledgment of the child's inner experience, with a determination to promote more adaptive function. This holds true for parents dealing with threats of suicide or self-injury, just as it does for other expressions of the child's anxiety or distress.

Rather than adopting these stances, the therapist should attempt to promote a supportive stance on the part of the child, which can best be described by the following parental message:

I will do anything in the world to protect you from harm—without giving in to threats.

What this attitude achieves, through the words, and more importantly through the parental behaviors described later, is a disassociation between parents' assessment of risk or manipulation and the action they take. The idea that if the child is genuinely at risk the parents' actions should be abandoned, but if the child is merely "bluffing," then that bluff should be called, is akin to the mistaken attitude we described in other sessions about coping with anxiety. In other words, just as the parents continue the SPACE Program despite the child being *really afraid*, they can maintain progress whether the child is truly threatening self-harm. The key is in protecting the child from harm while still promoting function. This can be done in various ways, and below are the two we have found to be most helpful.

Supportive Strategy I—Round-the-Clock Protection with the Help of Supporters

This strategy depends on the use of supporters and should follow or include the *Session Module on recruiting and engaging supporters*. Parents will create a supervision schedule to prevent any harm to the child. The three goals of this strategy are to:

1. Protect the child by creating supervision and minimizing opportunity for self-harm.
2. Support the child through the presence and caring of parents and others.
3. Minimize the likelihood of future threats by avoiding reinforcement of the threat.

Inform the Child of Parental Decision
Parents should calmly inform children that the threats they have made to harm themselves are very serious. They should explain that it is their job as parents to prevent any harm coming to the children, even from themselves. Parents should state the amount of time the supervision will last (to be decided with the therapist based on threat assessment; at least one whole day) and should explain that they will have help from others in keeping the child safe.

As in all SPACE Program steps, the parents should present their intention calmly and avoid any argument or provocation. The decision should be presented as a foregone conclusion and should not be debated. If children state there is no need for supervision as they are not going to act on the threat, parents should acknowledge this but explain they must take precautions after such a threat has been made.

> What you said earlier, about killing yourself, is very serious. We love you very much and as your parents it is always our job to keep you safe. We will do anything we can to make sure you do not get hurt, even from yourself. We have decided that we must supervise you to make sure nothing bad happens to you. We will watch you for 24 hours and then decide how to proceed. Because we need to keep you absolutely safe we will get help from relatives or friends who care about you and will help us to protect you. For the next 24 hours you will not be alone. This is not a punishment and you should definitely tell us if you think about suicide so that we can help you to stay safe and get better.

Create Supervision Schedule
The therapist helps the parents to create a supervision schedule for the child. The supervision schedule should ensure that the child is never left

alone for the full time that the supervision is in effect. Even if a parent is able to be at home the entire time with the child, the help of other supporters should be recruited. This will allow the child to feel the care of more than only the parents and may create opportunities for a healthier dialogue mediated by the supporters.

The closeness of the supervision should be determined based on the level of threat and age of the children. In all cases, children should be prevented from locking themselves in any room without a supporter present, including bedroom and bathroom. If the child is allowed to leave the house, a supervisor should be within eyesight at all times. If the worry is particularly great, the child should not be alone in a room for more than a very brief time. If the supervision in incompatible with other activities the child would normally engage in, such as going to classes or visiting friends, these activities should be cancelled. The explanation to the child should be that "Right now, the most important thing is to keep you safe."

Supervision—Not Punishment
The therapist should ensure that the parents and all additional supporters understand that the goal of the supervision is not to punish the child for having made the threat. Children express distress in many ways and for many reasons, and should not experience the parental need to protect them as recrimination. Although many children will not like the supervision, and may voice the sentiment that they feel punished, the actual emotional experience will be determined by the behavior of the parents and supporters. Arguments about the need for supervision or its details should be avoided altogether, and the parents should simply meet all such arguments with the statement: "This is what we believe we need to do right now to keep you safe." This should be repeated no more than once every few hours, and all other invitations to debate should be declined with silence.

Supporters should allow the child to engage in activities that do not pose a risk and should only interact with the child to the degree that they are invited to do so. Some children may choose to talk with them or spend the time together while others will prefer to ignore their presence most of the time. The rule should be to remember that their role is to create protection for children because they care about them. Lecturing, in particular, should be discouraged as it will convince the child that the real purpose is not one of protection but rather a form of punishment or retaliation. If the child chooses to engage supporters in conversation, this is a positive thing (if it does not include primarily debate about the necessity of the supervision). Supporters should express their care for the children and support for the steps the parents are taking in helping them to overcome anxiety. The supporters can offer their help in any way and suggest that rather than talking about suicide, children may come to them when feeling particularly distressed. When children state that it is only the parents' actions that have prompted their threats to themselves, the supporters should explain that the parents have no choice but to try to help children overcome the anxiety. Supporters can attempt to engage children in the process of overcoming the anxiety disorder by explaining that if they were more cooperative they would have a greater degree of control over the process (for example, in determining the rate of change or the specific target goals addressed).

After Supervision

When the supervision schedule is complete, parents, in appropriate consultation with the therapist, determine whether the home can return to more routine functioning. If so, the parents should state simply to the child that they now feel able to do so and that they will continue to fulfill their roles as parents as best they can.

Supportive Strategy II—ER Visit

A visit to the emergency room (ER) can be a positive experience, if parents convey love and concern as the reason for going. The three goals of this strategy are:

1. Provide immediate protection and risk assessment.
2. Convey concern without acquiescing to stopping the SPACE Program process.
3. Minimize the likelihood of future threats by avoiding reinforcement of the threat.

Although visiting the ER because of threats of violence to one's self is commonly done immediately following the threat, this does not have to

232

be exclusively the case. Parents who are concerned about threats a child previously made can choose to seek emergency psychiatric attention if they consider the child still to be at risk.

The therapist can help the parents to present the decision to visit the ER to the child as the natural outcome of his self-directed threats. "*When you say you will kill yourself, we have no choice but to take you to the hospital.*" In most cases of suicidal statements triggered by parents resisting the anxiety, the child will respond to the decision with a retraction of the threatening statement. Many children encourage the parents to go to the hospital, up until the point at which they realize that is actually what is happening. Once the decision to go to the ER has been made and expressed to the child, the parents should complete the visit despite the child's retractions. This will serve two purposes: First, it will allow for a real assessment to be made rather than relying on the child's shifting attitude. Second, it will help the child to understand that, once made, suicidal threats cannot easily be unmade—thereby encouraging more careful deliberation in the future. Parents should simply repeat: "We understand, but it's our job to make sure"; or "I hear you but I love you too much to just ignore what you said."

Throughout the process, including the trip to the hospital, the visit there and the time that follows, parents should be encouraged to maintain a calm and nonpunitive attitude. Visiting the ER reflects the need for emergency medical attention, and is not a tool for punishment or threat. After the visit, parents should avoid threatening the child with repeated visits in the future.

- By maintaining a loving and supportive stance, while avoiding either giving in to the threats or exacerbating them, parents will usually be able to minimize the use of such threats in the future and allow for more progress in overcoming the anxiety.

CHAPTER THIRTEEN

Increasing Collaboration Between Parents

A child's anxiety disorder has the potential to affect not only the healthy boundaries between parent and child but can also place considerable stress on other family-system dynamics. Parents' ability to cooperate collaboratively between themselves as well as dilemmas relating to additional children in the family are examples of the broader challenges facing the family.

Key points in this chapter:

- Challenges to collaboration between parents of anxious children.
- Improving parents' ability to work collaboratively.
- When one parent refuses to cooperate.
- Dealing with sibling issues.

COLLABORATION BETWEEN PARENTS

The relationship between parental conflict and childhood anxiety is well documented and intuitively sensible (Manassis & Hood, 1998; Messer & Beidel, 1994). Most of the research into this association has focused on the ways in which elevated frequency and severity of conflict (Davies & Cummings, 1994; Grych & Fincham, 1990), or less productive mechanisms of settling arguments can augment a child's anxiety and impede adjustment (Cummings, Ballard, El-Sheikh, & Lake, 1991). In particular, arguments that relate directly to the child, such as disagreements about child-rearing practices, have the potential to trigger or exacerbate anxiety in children (Dadds & Powell, 1991). In the context of a child's anxiety disorder this describes a vicious cycle. The presence of a child with an anxiety disorder can highlight parental disagreement and aggravate discord that otherwise might be less explicit. For instance, an anxious child's demands for reassurance or attempts to control family schedule might trigger arguments over the degree of firmness or flexibility that parents should display. In turn, the parental dissent that would otherwise be less prominent, further increases the child's anxiety, creating even more cause for quarrel between the parents.

Parents of anxious children, particularly those who disagree over the correct response to the child's anxiety, will also often become ensnared in an unproductive "blame-game." Each parent blames the other for creating the problem, or for preventing its solution. Sometimes parents will be reluctant to continue the process of coping supportively with the children's anxiety, because of a sense that their partner is acting in a way that is harmful rather than helpful. In therapy such a parent might express the feeling that, "as long as she continues to act this way there is no point in coming to these sessions." This "resigning" weakens both parents' ability to support the anxious child and confronts the therapist with a seemingly impossible situation. Even when parents choose to disengage for more innocuous reasons, such as lack of time or the desire to avoid confrontation, their abdication has the effect of weakening the therapeutic process.

Even partial improvement in the degree of cooperation and collaboration between parents can cause significant enhancement to their ability to promote better functioning in the child. When this occurs, a reverse cycle can be created where partial collaboration leads to improvement in the child's symptoms, less cause for argument, and greater emotional well-being for the family system overall. As the child experiences the rift between parents shrinking rather than widening, the emotional stress is diminished and confidence in the parents' ability to provide support is increased.

Although solving parental conflict while treating the child's anxiety can seem like a daunting task, the therapist should keep in mind that it is not necessary for the parents to reach complete agreement; decreasing the degree of conflict, particularly surrounding practical issues such as how to respond to the child, is often enough to allow for great improvement. Similarly to the approach we take in working with the child, we recommend treating partial improvement in parents' working alliance as highly valuable. In our work with parents we do not strive for complete solutions to their problems as a couple (if such a thing exists), or for unanimous agreement about their parental roles. In fact, requiring total resolution of family or marital conflict, as a condition for improving a child's anxiety or parental functioning, is actually counterproductive. Insisting on perfect harmony as a condition for parent guidance will hamper improvement by creating an impossible prerequisite to positive action. In fact, by allowing for partial improvement, parents can model a more productive strategy for the child as well. Just as the child need not completely overcome anxiety before taking on partial challenges, the parents do not have to achieve total resolution before undertaking positive parental steps. Sometimes even a tiny reduction in the rift between the parents can be experienced as enormous by the child.

Typical Rifts Between Parents

Mark: "Ever since Alan was small, his mother's spoiled him. She does everything for him. She doesn't even let him make his own bed! How does she expect him to grow up when she is so protective? When he wanted to go to a sleepover at a friend's house, she almost didn't let him go. And then she called him 10 times over the course of the evening. She's the one with anxiety issues! If she'd only let him, he'd learn to cope on his own. When I was his age I was going to work with my dad after school to help support the family, and here he is, at the same age, sleeping in our bed half the time!"

Dina: "He doesn't understand that the world is a different place now. Today children need to be children. They need to be protected from all the dangers lurking outside, and to be allowed to grow up at their own pace. He wants his boy to 'be a man' like him. What does he want? For our kid to grow up and hate us?; To break his spirit?; For him to end up losing it completely?"

Pete: "The kid hardly leaves her room. Doesn't get together with friends, doesn't talk on the phone, doesn't do anything! And her mother just lets her. She makes no demands. On the contrary, she lets it go on day after day. If I was at home, things would have changed long ago."

Sandy: "It's easy for him. Sure, he comes home in the evening, eats, watches TV, and goes to bed. I'd like to see him dealing with this girl for just one day. What does he think? That I don't want to help her? That I haven't already tried everything? I need to get through day after day with this child, who is afraid of the entire world. Let me go out to work, and let him try and help her, if he's so smart. It's real easy to criticize someone else!"

Norris: "This boy is just like me. I get him. At his age I also had lots of fears. I used to worry about everyone: my parents, my friends, I even worried about our dog! I was sure that if I did something wrong, or even if I had a bad thought, our poor dog would get run over by a car. I couldn't sleep at night. I was afraid to be alone. So, my son is the same way. It's probably genetic. When he started in with his thoughts and strange habits, I sat down with him right away and told him I know all about it. That the world really is a scary place, and there's nothing to be ashamed of. In the end I got over it and so will he, in time. There's nothing to make a fuss about. If my wife had fears like that she would understand, but she can't get inside his head."

Leslie: "First of all, he definitely did not get over it! He's still full of fears, and his day is full of rituals because of them. Don't say this, and don't do that, and if anything is moved out of its place it's a disaster. I love my husband, and I accept him, but why should I let him transfer all his fears on to our child?"

The first couple, Mark and Dina, have different ideas about raising children: Mark believes in making clear demands and exposing children to the world. Dina believes in giving them a pleasant environment while protecting and sheltering them. These are natural differences, and many children grow up perfectly well in spite of similar differences of opinion between their parents. But when a child has an anxiety disorder and his parents have to take action to address it, this kind of difference can cause a growing rift. Their son Alan has learned that if he magnifies his distress signals the gulf between his parents will grow, allowing him more leeway for avoidance.

Pete and Sandy's case exemplifies a more mundane cause of differences between parents: time! Most couples in the early 21st century do not spend equal amounts of time with their children, or take equal responsibility for the day-to-day management of child needs and roles (Bianchi, 2000; Guryan, Hurst, Kearney, & National Bureau of Economic Research, 2008). Sandy, who spends most of the day with her daughter, feels exhausted and worn out. She does not believe that Pete understands this, because he has to contend much less often with the difficulties she faces every day. This is a common disparity; mothers typically spend more time at home, and even when the father is home, many children come to their mother first, with most of their problems or worries. Further amplifying the problem is that mothers and fathers often disagree about just how much time their partner is actually spending with the children (Coley & Morris, 2002). In such a situation it is not surprising that tension and tempers can run high. Sandy's remark—that things would be different if Pete had to deal with their daughter on a daily basis—expresses the difficult reality of many mothers.

Norris and Leslie's argument demonstrates another frequent cause of discord between parents: differential identification with the child's anxious experience. Norris feels that only he can "get in his son's head" and understand him, while Leslie feels that Norris is causing his own problems to be replicated in their child. Which of the two of them is more entitled to determine the parental attitude toward the child? **One parent asks: "How can you help him when you have no idea what he's going through?", and the other replies: "How can you help him when you're exactly like him?"**

The therapist cannot realistically expect any of these couples to completely agree on a single position. The hope that one parent will suddenly realize that the other has been right all along, and change his or her attitude accordingly, is a fantasy. Moreover, the attempts to change someone's mind, usually characterized by criticism or laying of blame, causes further resistance. But it is possible to bring the couple closer, to improve the parental boundary and shape a supportive stance, in spite of the differences in parental attitudes.

Bringing Opposites Closer

Roy grew up in a large family, with parents who believed in a strict upbringing and in discipline. He is striving to implement the same approach with his own children. He disciplines them, enforces clear boundaries, and punishes when necessary. Della, on the other hand, grew up in a home where openness and democracy were paramount. She believes children thrive in an open and liberal atmosphere, and that words such as *no* and *forbidden* only depress their young spirits, which need to grow and flourish. Roy and Della have always had these differences, but with their two older children they seemed able to balance them successfully. They would even tease each other over their differences. Ever since Emma, their youngest, was born 7 years ago, the arguments between them have been incessant. Emma is a worrisome and anxious child, who draws the little confidence she has from her closeness to her parents. Roy feels that she is spoiled, bossy, and lacking in boundaries, while Della feels that Roy is too cold and unbending toward their daughter. She accuses him of expecting all children to be the same, and of being unwilling to accept their child's weaknesses. In a meeting with their therapist the following statements were made:

DELLA: Why is he so strict?

THERAPIST: How would you like him to be? What about him would you like to change?

DELLA: I'd like him to show Emma that he understands her, that he accepts her.

THERAPIST: You feel that under the current circumstances you are the only one who understands her?

DELLA: Precisely. That's why I have to be as close and tender as possible. Sometimes I would also like to put some limits, but then I think about how it's only from me that she gets any warmth and understanding, and I have to be flexible.

THERAPIST: How about you, Roy? How would you like Della to act?

ROY: Unfortunately, in our home I am the only one who sees how things really are, the only one setting any boundaries.

THERAPIST: If Della set more limits, would you be able to relax your attitude a little?

ROY: If only she would! If she would take responsibility sometimes, I could stop being the "bad guy" all the time!

In this case Roy and Della are actually much closer to cooperating than they realize. They both long to escape from their all-embracing attitudes. Della would like to be able to set limits sometimes, and Roy longs to feel free to express the warmth he feels toward his daughter. But when each wants more than anything for the other to accept his or her position, the result is paradoxical. The desire to convince and persuade causes the opposite result in the other parent. The more one parent presses for flexibility, the more demanding the other becomes. This is because that parent believes that they alone represents the functional demands of the real world. And conversely, the more demanding one parent becomes, the more accommodating the other feels they needs to be.

Obviously, parents are not actually "demanding" or "protective," as these are simplistic and reductive descriptions that do not capture the conflicting motivations and natural ambivalence that are usually central to experiencing most dilemmas. Parents who appear to be overly protective may also have an inner voice clamoring for the ability to set clearer boundaries, and in the demanding parent is often hidden a comforting and compassionate voice. This assumption echoes a similar one with regard to the conflicted motivations of the anxious child. Alongside the voices insisting on avoidance, there is also the will to face anxiety and overcome it.

In working with parents, the therapist tries to help them to shape their responses to the child in such a way as to amplify and support the healthy voices within the child. In addressing parental conflict and disagreement, the therapist tries to help parents to recognize the complexity and heterogeneity in themselves and in each other. This belief in multiple "inner voices" in parents is reinforced by conversations with them, and when the therapist is sensitive and respectful of both parents, they can bring these voices to the surface. Seemingly protective parents will communicate their desire for clearer boundaries and better coping if they do not feel embattled and defensive, or as though expressing this desire would be an admission of having been wrong all along. A putatively demanding parent can express the desire for a warm and close relationship with the child. For the hidden voices to be expressed the parents need to receive recognition of the legitimacy of their dominant position. On the other hand, if the parents feel that their overall position is being attacked, they will usually respond by becoming more entrenched and polarized.

Barbara found it hard to go to work, because her 12-year-old daughter Iris had become very afraid of remaining home alone. She cut back on the hours she spent at work, but still missed many workdays because of Iris's anxiety attacks. Rafi, her husband, accused Barbara of making Iris worse with her overprotectiveness. He also criticized her for not taking her job seriously, and said she would eventually get herself fired. As expected, his resolute demands only made Barbara angrier and more fixed in her position. Iris, who felt threatened by her father, grew apart from him.

Their therapist assumed that other voices also resided in each of the parents. He was convinced that Barbara longed to ease the burden of Iris's never-ending demands, and that Rafi missed the warm relationship he used to have with his daughter. However, Barbara could not vocalize her hidden desire. Had she admitted, or even implied that she would like to be able to stand up better to Iris's demands, Rafi would have immediately pounced: "But that is what I'm always saying! Do you see? Even you admit I'm right!" Rafi was in a similar bind: He was afraid that if he expressed how much he missed Iris, Barbara would blame the rift on him and accuse him of betraying his duty as a father. To break free of this vicious cycle of mutual negativity, the therapist suggested a meeting with special rules. The meeting would be divided in two. During the first part he would talk with Rafi, with Barbara present but not involved. She would be allowed only to listen, even if she felt that the things said were absolutely wrong. In the second part the roles would be reversed, and Rafi would be the one to listen silently while the therapist talked with Barbara. Both parents agreed to these rules. In this manner the therapist hoped to create an environment in which parents could express their hidden voice without interruption from the other spouse. When talking with Rafi, the therapist emphasized that his role is necessary, but thankless. As the representative of "reality," Rafi felt that if he lessened his demands, even just by a little, he would be paving the way for avoidance and deterioration. This is a difficult and frustrating job, because as the "bad guy" he became the focus of Iris's hostility. The therapist asked Rafi if he ever felt like acting differently, like letting go of the bad guy job and getting close to his daughter again. Rafi answered that that was what he wanted more than anything. When the therapist asked him if he believes Iris misses him, too, his eyes filled with tears. The therapist ended his session with Rafi by saying that perhaps it would be possible for them to resume their previous closeness, especially if Rafi were not the only one responsible for "reality." During the course of the talk with Rafi, Barbara tried to interrupt, but the therapist politely stopped her. He began his time with her by emphasizing her maternal feelings, which did not allow her to ignore her daughter's suffering. Then he asked her about the difficult steps along the way, where she slowly gave up her personal life to support and protect Iris. He asked whether there was ever a moment when she wished for a different relationship with Iris. Barbara expressed her longing for a bit of time for herself. She said she missed feeling like a person, as well as a mother. The therapist, who believed the couple's relationship was basically sound in spite of their difficulties, asked whether Iris's problem had impinged on their activities as a couple. Barbara said she would love to be able to go out with Rafi alone, as a couple again, even for a short while. The therapist summed things up:

"I am convinced you are both parents with deep parental feelings, and you are both right about a lot of things in your different attitudes. You, Barbara, feel that Iris needs closeness and warmth, in order to build up her confidence in life. Otherwise, you feel she is hopeless. You plead persistently with Rafi to understand this, and to give her what she needs. You, Rafi, feel that if Iris is not faced with the demands of reality, she will get steadily worse. You beg, and sometimes pressure Barbara to under-stand this, and to go in this direction. Both things are indispensable, but at the moment you are accomplishing the opposite of what you want. Rafi, when you pressure Barbara she feels that she is the only one giving Iris love and warmth, and she intensifies her forgiveness and protection. And when you, Barbara, plead with Rafi, he feels like the only realistic one, and then he has no choice but to toughen his demands. So you are each causing your spouse to act in the opposite way to what you actually want.

Furthermore, you, Rafi, criticize Barbara, are angry with Iris, and thus increase the distance between you and your daughter. This must be the last thing you want. And you, Barbara, feel cornered, that you cannot limit Iris's demands, and that you are giving up your life, as a person and as a couple. But this cannot work. You giving up your life will not make things better for Iris—it will make them worse. I suggest that in our meetings we make a plan so Iris can experience the two of you closer together, instead of further apart. We will plan days when everyone goes easier on Iris, and also plan more focused demands, which you will both make. And we won't forget about you as a couple: If you don't have a life together as a couple, you are abandoning Iris! I will stop any one of you who tries to return to your old tune! I'm sure Iris will benefit, and so will you!"

This statement laid down the foundations that were needed for the parents to begin cooperating. Rafi was able to grow closer to Iris, and Barbara didn't miss work anymore. And Iris began gradually showing signs of adjusting.

Concealment and Cooperation

Fifteen-year-old Dan suffered from panic attacks at school, characterized by shortness of breath, elevated heart rate, and tremors. Dan was very fearful of losing control of himself and acting inappropriately. He was terrified during the attacks but also constantly apprehensive between attacks that another one might be imminent. Whenever Dan felt he might have a panic attack he would call his parents to come take him home. After consulting the therapist, his parents, David and Martha, decided not to come get him in the middle of the school day any more. When Dan called, they would remind him that he has to stay in school, and that he can go to the counselor's office until he's calmed down. The school counselor was involved in the plan, and Dan had free access to her office, even when she was not there. Two days after they explained this plan to Dan, he called his mother from school and said he was on the verge of panic. Martha told herself that she needs to treat the call as an opportunity to set healthier parental boundaries and said:

"Dan, I know this is difficult but I'm sure you can cope. If you have to, go to the counselor's room and call me from there in 15 minutes. Bye." With great difficulty she hung up the phone.

Dan immediately dialed his father:

"D-D-Dad . . . I . . . I . . . I don't know what's happening to me! I can't breathe . . . I think . . . I think it's serious . . . I'm choking . . . I—I—I . . . "

"Dan, I'm on my way!" his father responded immediately.

Only on his way to the school, did David recall the counselor's office and the plan they had made. Dan's anxiety overwhelmed his personal boundary, and caused him to race to the school. On their way home in the car David turned around to Dan and told him: "Just don't tell your Mom I picked you up. She'll never let us forget it."

David's impulse to rush to Dan's aid was understandable. Hearing your son gasping for air over the telephone is enough to make almost anyone lose their cool. The decision to keep the event secret from Martha, together with Dan, is a more serious mistake. The alliance created between himself and his son by saying "Don't tell Mom!" will inevitably weaken the parental boundary and portray the father as more closely allied with anxiety than with the forces striving for health.

The therapist, confronted with this kind of miscommunication, can help parents to resume healthier collaboration, improving the child's likelihood of adhering to the plan in the future. Even a negative event such as the one described earlier could be utilized by the clinician as an opportunity to strengthen the parental collaboration. In this case the therapist advised the parents to enter the child's room together and to say to him:

We made a mistake today, and did not show our faith in your ability to cope with your anxiety. We have thought it through, and realize how wrong we were. In the future we will act differently. We will help you by reminding you of what you can do when you are feeling stressed, and will not help your anxiety by taking you home.

In this way the parents can signal to the child that the bond between them is strengthening, rather than the rift separating them growing. The failure becomes a reminder of the continuing parental commitment. The parents model to the child that errors and missteps need not mean that you stop trying. Both parents, not only the one admitting his mistake, need to be aware of the opportunity to turn this into a positive opportunity. This understanding can increase parents' ability to share mistakes with the spouse, and can make the other parent more accepting of errors.

Setting Aside a Time for Communication

Maintaining healthy parental boundaries requires continuous coordination, and it is usually best to set aside specific times to regularly discuss, plan, and coordinate responses to events. Things which go unsaid over the course of the day can be spoken about during the times set aside expressly for that purpose. Once the course of therapy or parent training is over, it is smart for parents to plan at least weekly meetings, which they can use for updating each other, coordinating, reevaluating, and making further decisions. These meetings improve parental efficiency greatly. They signal that the parents are engaged in a collaborative effort, and are working carefully and cautiously to rebuild their boundary, rather than relying on spontaneous reactions, which in the past did not prove to be effective in resolving the issues.

The meetings have a number of advantages. The first is improving communications between the parents. Constant communication is a basic condition for the existence of healthy family boundaries. Specifically allocating time for communication helps to battle another unfortunate tendency that many parents will encounter. This is the tendency to only talk about problems when they are causing the most stress and need to be solved right away. Like the debtor who only thinks about saving money when the bank calls, but soon goes back to imprudent spending, many parents will talk about the anxiety only when the child is acutely anxious or requires immediate attention. This ensures that communication will be centered on "putting out fires," rather than on longer-term strategies and also sets the stage for more negative attributions between parents. It is an unfortunate but familiar fact that people's ability to adopt the point of view of others is minimized under stress and tension. By talking about the problem at a predetermined time, parents may be able to achieve much greater meetings of the minds, as well as having the leeway to plan further ahead.

Another advantage of specifically allocating time for discussion is in preventing situations in which the parents find themselves arguing about the child's anxiety right in front of the child, in real time. Such arguments can be reduced significantly by postponing them to the prearranged discussion time. Instead of getting swept up into an argument, one of the parents can remind the other: "Let's leave this for our talk!" Anxious children, just like all others, are very good at recognizing disparity between their parents. Arresting an argument before it can develop, saying "This is for the discussion between us!" tells them that their parents are concerned with maintaining their union, and focused on working together. This message, rather than exacerbating children's anxiety by highlighting the disagreement between the parents, gives them a feeling of security created when they encounter a more united front.

Setting aside regular times for discussion and coordination presents parents with an opportunity to plan restorative actions, such as the one described earlier in Dan's case. And finally, postponing discussions for later helps to keep disagreements between the parents from escalating. Parents of anxious children often ascribe far-reaching blame on each other's mistakes: "Now you've ruined everything!," "There's no point going on with you—I give up!" This type of remark, made in anger, can cause severe counterreactions. Parental agreements, reached after difficult labor, can fall apart in one loud argument. The act of delaying the discussion can turn a fight into a fruitful dialogue.

Tempering the Accusations

The therapist working with the parents of an anxious child should be aware that when parents blame each other for the child's anxiety, they make those issues worse, *even if there is some truth in their accusations*. The pattern of blame can, in and of itself, turn a positive understanding into a negative process. The damage that laying blame causes stems from its impact on the parents' actions, on their relationship as a couple, and on the child's experience.

Attributing blame heralds a process of marginalization. Either the accused parents are shoved to the side and become neutralized and banished from involvement because of their "mistakes," or the parents who feel that only they understand the problem push themselves away and become what we have sometimes termed *Right but all alone*. Sometimes, through the exchange of accusations and the allocation of blame a parent can feel at once both marginalized and right but all alone.

Right but all alone are the parents who have lost their power to influence the goings-on in their family, but feel that they can see all the mistakes their spouse is making. Although their perceptions may hold some truth, they can do nothing to improve the situation. Their insights are perceived only as criticisms and accusations. Even if the other parents feel there is truth in the things being said, instead of feeling support they feel the opposite. Their only desire is to keep the accusing parent away and neutralize their criticisms. This makes the other parents lonelier still. Their only consolation is in being right more and more of the time. Sometimes they even boast about how differently the child behaves around them, which only deepens the frustration the accused parent feels, and widens the rift between the couple.

Therapists are often implicitly or explicitly invited to take sides in these situations. But by doing so, they put their own ability to remain effective at risk. In our work we have encountered parents who attempt to align themselves with the therapist, even suggesting that they have "brought their spouse in" so the therapist can "tell them the facts." In other words their only hope is to hear the therapist echoing what they believe to be the truth. For the therapist, accepting an invitation of this kind means propagating the existing family dynamic in which parents feel they hold the key to knowledge and understanding while the other parents feel misunderstood and blamed. Rather, the therapist should strive to create an atmosphere that will allow both parents to recognize the value of each other's point of view, as well as reminding them of their shared goals and common objectives.

The therapist might feel challenged by the recognition of the truth in what an accusing parent says. One might ask: "But what if the other parent **really is** to blame for the child's problem?" However, this kind of conceptualization is always overly simplistic and incomplete. Anxiety is the result of many processes, including a physiological tendency to strong emotional and physical reactions, outside circumstances that aggravate these tendencies (such as a frightening or traumatic experience, or sudden changes in life's circumstances), a diminishment of the child's or the family's resources and coping (due to the child's or a parent's illness, financial straits, changes in the parents' presence in the home, etc.), establishment of circumstances that allow avoidance (for example, truancy, isolation, cessation of routine activities), the parents' difficulties in coordinating between themselves, or arguments between them, and others. Even if one of the parents is a major contributor to the process, they are not "to blame" for the child's anxiety. However, by moderating the patterns of accusations and the reactions they trigger, the therapist can help to create conditions in which both parents can cope much better.

This is why we consider tempering the parents' mutual accusations to be a mission of utmost importance for therapists. They should explain to the parents that the accusatory stance perpetuates the problem, and thereby pulls the rug from under the very accusations made. The therapist emphasizes that there is no way for one parent to be solely responsible for the child's difficulties. It may be helpful to remind the accusing parents that it is a fantasy to expect the other parents to "confess their guilt" and change deeply held attitudes in accordance with their expectations. In fact, the very attempt to make them do so reinforces precisely the most problematic sides of each parent's position. The therapist should strive to achieve a limited and practical cooperation between the parents even when many of their fundamental beliefs do not match. A partial and practical cooperation can be positively reflected in the child's experience. Children, discovering that their anxious reactions now cause their parents to come closer together instead of pushing them farther apart, begin to experience a parental boundary, which introduces some stability and structure into their life. It is important to remember that a part of the child is eager to cope with their anxiety. The cooperation between their parents, even if it is partial and limited, strengthens this part of the child, and supports them.

Alice and Terry's 11-year-old son Manny suffers from a panic disorder with agoraphobia. Since early childhood Manny has exhibited a tendency to various fears and anxieties, and many compulsive rituals. Because of his fear of his panic attacks, and because he believes these attacks are very dangerous to him, Manny refuses to be alone, even momentarily. He never knows when he will believe he needs immediate medical attention, and all the doctors' attempts to convince him he is healthy have failed. Alice is Manny's primary caregiver, and she goes to great lengths to calm him in any way possible. She spends almost all her time with him, other than the few hours when he is in school. She has gone with him for extensive medical check-ups dozens of times over the years, and because of his difficulties she even gave up on her plan to return to work after years as a stay-at-home mom.

Terry has felt for years that Alice's treatment of Manny is very wrong. He has tried on numerous occasions to explain to her that her repeated attempts to calm Manny do not work, and that he needs to be allowed to feel "like a normal child." Time after time he has watched Alice give in to Manny's demands that she stop whatever she is doing and come to him, take him to a doctor again, or just be with him. Terry believes many of Manny's fears are a manipulation meant to gain him complete control over his mother's time, and he is angry that she doesn't see that. He blames Alice for Manny being so limited today that he cannot even leave the house alone, go to friends, on school trips, or just live a normal life because of his fears, and in Terry's opinion these are direct consequences of Alice's bad decisions. Furthermore, he sees how Manny uses his fears to get what he wants, or to shirk responsibilities. When it's time for him to go to bed, for example, he starts complaining that he can't breathe in the bedroom, and so has to stay in the living room, where he can watch TV, of course. "You're ruining the child," Terry says to Alice time and again, but she believes that it is impossible to just ignore Manny's obvious distress. Her heart wrenches every time she hears Terry's words. "How can he blame this on me?" she asks. Alice acknowledges that there is some truth in what Terry is saying, and that Manny is usually better behaved with him. But his criticisms serve only to make her feel weaker and more hopeless.

After a few meetings, during which he listened to what Alice and Terry had to say, the therapist addressed the issue:

Alice and Terry,

I have been listening to you over the course of our last meetings, and I sympathized sometimes with your pain, Alice, and sometimes with yours, Terry. The entire time I identified with what you have in common, with the parenting principle, which rises above all the differences between you, the concern you both have for your son, and the effort you invest in him. You do not have an easy child, and you have both already done so much, and continue to do so much to help him.

You, Alice, have sacrificed years of your life to taking care of your special child, whose needs are much greater than most children's. You have given him everything: your time, your energy, your worry, and your love. There has been no sacrifice you were not willing to make, nothing you were not willing to give up for him. I see and appreciate your effort, and believe you deserve not only my total respect, but everyone's. But in spite of all your effort, you have not been able to mitigate his suffering. You were willing to be his "security blanket," even at the cost of other central things in your life, and yet he still felt insecure. You told me how Manny sometimes says that he cannot breathe, that he has no air. I think you, too, for years now have had no air. You have long since stopped taking any air for yourself, but you have not been able to give him the air you gave up.

Terry, to you I want to say how much I appreciate the way you think about Manny's problem. Time after time you analyzed the problem precisely and in depth, and said some of the same things I was planning to say. I think that you also experience a lot of frustration. You feel that you understand what needs to be done to change the situation, but in spite of your efforts in that direction, the situation remains unchanged.

I think the time has come for you both to make a change. All your efforts so far have not produced an improvement. Something in your good intentions has gone awry. You, Alice, wanted to provide security, but Manny has become more and more dependent. You, Terry, wanted to convince Alice to be less protective, but your remarks were taken as criticisms. So instead of fortifying Alice, you weaken her. I would like to propose a new system for the two of you to try. I suggest that you, Alice, take back some of the air you deserve. You will need support in order to do this. And I recommend that we make a plan together that will ensure you get the support you need. If you cannot breathe, Manny will continue to suffocate for many years to come. If you cannot live your life, Manny will have no life of his own. And to you, Terry, I say that in a place where words don't help, they need to be replaced with actions. When you know what needs to be done, do it! When you understand what actions need to be taken, take them! Don't wait for Alice to be convinced. You have a lot of wisdom. Instead of trying to bestow it on Alice, use it. Instead of being Alice's teacher, or preacher, be her husband, her helpmate, be her support sometimes! I am sure that if you do that, then she will also be able to act, because we will provide her with the conditions to do so. You will both feel yourselves getting stronger. Not only that, but you will soon see how strong Manny can also be, in a positive way, and not just in a negative way.

Attaining Limited Cooperation

It will often appear as though improving the parents' whole relationship, or completely bridging the differences in their attitudes and styles, is a necessary precondition for them to be able to cooperate with regard to their anxious child. Many therapists become embroiled in this feeling, and some will send parents to lengthy couples' therapy before agreeing to intervene around the child's anxiety. But total agreement on ideals and parenting styles is not usually a feasible goal, and getting caught up in an "all or nothing" conceptualization will waste precious time and energy, often only making the situation worse. Experience has shown us that in most cases a complete solution to the couples' problems is not imperative for working on the anxiety. Presenting it as such could ensure that the situation does not improve for a long time.

In the beginning of this chapter we described the story of Roy and Della, whose differing parenting attitudes had become a source of conflict when they faced the difficulties dealing with their daughter Emma's anxiety. They chose to begin the process of change by making one small joint decision:

> Roy and Della decided they would no longer give in to Emma's request that her older brother sleep in her room when she's anxious. In spite of the differences of opinion between them they agreed that this request was not fair on the brother, who had lately begun expressing his impatience with the situation. On the first night it was Roy, as usual, who refused the request. Emma immediately turned to her mother and asked her to revoke the decision. Della was about to agree when her eyes met Roy's and she recalled their joint decision. She said: "Dad and I decided that's not such a good idea." The ensuing argument was short, and when it was over Emma slept alone. This event foretold the possibility of a new "family dance" for the three of them; one in which the parents display a limited, but solid, cooperation regarding practical decisions, in spite of their continued disagreement on the principal issues and their varied levels of identification with Emma's suffering.

Role Play—Switching Places

One technique the therapist can use to increase flexibility in parental attitudes and foster this kind of limited cooperation when parents are clinging to opposing poles, is role play. For a limited period of time, each parent assumes the other's role in the specific area in which they are trying to achieve cooperation. For instance, the parent who is most accommodating assumes the role of "accommodation-guard" in the area in question, responsible for identifying accommodation and helping to prevent it. Meanwhile, the parent who has stood for stricter demands and boundaries takes responsibility for making the child feel better. The exercise is time-limited to minimize the parent's apprehensions and both parents commit to not commenting or criticizing the other, even if they feel they are not staying "in role."

Adele and Steve, the parents of 7-year-old Shelly, chose to role play regarding Shelly's habit of asking for reassurance whenever she was troubled by a worrisome thought. Every evening, when it started to grow dark, Shelly would be besieged by worries about her health, and that of the rest of the family. She would ask endless questions like, "How do you know I won't have a heart attack"; "How can you be sure the food we ate wasn't spoiled?"; "How would you know if you had cancer?" Adele and Steve would start by answering her questions, but they never seemed to end, going on for hours at a time. Steve would try to get her to think about something else, or to resist answering but she would begin crying, begging them to answer "just one more thing." Steve didn't believe Shelly would ever break the habit on her own and tried to forbid her to ask any questions they had already answered in the past. Adele accused him of being heartless, and of being unaffected by his daughter's crying. She would open up books and go online to try to find answers that would put Shelly's mind at ease. Following their decision to role play for a few evenings, the nightly scenario changed dramatically. As expected, Shelly began with her usual questions. She said she had heard on TV about AIDS and wanted to understand whether she might have it. Adele spoke to her softly, but told her she must try to cope, that it is just her anxiety acting up, and that she is willing to come sit with her for a while but not to answer the questions because that doesn't really help. A very surprised Shelly became confused by this unexpected reaction. She was silent for a few moments, and then began crying miserably. At this point Steve sat down next to her and enveloped her in a warm embrace. "It must be terribly uncomfortable to have such scary thoughts in your head, right?" he asked, and Shelly clung to him tightly. In the end it was Steve who sat with her until she became calm again. At their meeting with the therapist the next day Adele and Steve could not contain their excitement. Steve spoke of the warmth he felt for Shelly as she snuggled in his arms, while Adele was awed by her own ability to withstand her automatic response to Shelly's distress.

WHEN ONE PARENT REFUSES TO BE PART OF THE TREATMENT

In some cases differing attitudes toward the problem or toward psychotherapy in general will preclude the active involvement of both parents in treatment. The therapist can work with one parent while actively working to maintain open lines of communication with the other. In some cases this can lead to the disengaged parent choosing to join the process at a later stage.

Accepting the Limitation

Sometimes the therapist may find it impossible to obtain the cooperation of one of the parents in the process of overcoming the child's anxiety. The refusal can stem from many reasons: mistrust; resistance to psychological treatment in general; a declared disbelief in the existence of a problem; lack of time; not identifying with the basic principles of the treatment; or the belief that the problem lies entirely with the other parent. In these situations the therapist may only be able to work with one parent and will need to help him or her to make unilateral changes, without the active support of the other parent.

When acting unilaterally, it is even more crucial for the therapist to avoid succumbing to a totalistic and overly simplistic view of the absent parent. Resisting, for example, statements that impute blame on the noncollaborative parents for the situation, or that imply that they will somehow sabotage any gains that are made. Such remarks, whether made by therapists or endorsed by them can only serve to further increase polarization and escalation. Therapists should remain cognizant of the fact that while their involvement is short termed, both parents will remain part of the equation for the long haul. The therapist should emphasize that anxiety is never caused by one parent, but that it is possible, even acting alone, to achieve some degree of improvement, thereby setting the stage for improved collaboration in the future.

Therapist and parent will need to face the realization that there are many aspects of life that are not directly controllable, despite the best of intentions. The parent cannot "force" the child to be less anxious or more motivated, and neither therapists nor parents can force an unwilling spouse to engage in treatment against their will or their values. Accepting the limits of one's influence is an expression of another kind of personal boundary. Acknowledging that each individual, even within couples, must make separate decisions and take the responsibility for them. In accepting this, the focus can shift away from the frustration of a noncollaborative partner and rest on what can actually be achieved. Any action taken with an acceptance of this personal boundary will be partial, and have limited goals. This allows the therapist to promote action even without the cooperation of both parents. Through limited, unilateral actions the statement can be made: "This is my position as a parent! I must act this way!" And in the same breath we are saying: "I cannot guarantee the success of my actions!"

Below are some principles that will aid the therapist in counseling the parent who chooses to act unilaterally to improve his or her coping with the child's problems, and to diminish any contribution to escalation and polarization between the parents.

Act, Don't Sermonize

One of the surest ways to escalate tensions between parents is lecturing and preaching to one of the parents. The parent on the receiving end of the lecture feels devalued, disrespected, and resentful of the other's patronizing attitude. In spite of all this, it is all too hard to break the lecturing habit, partially because the person doing it is not always aware of it. He or she may think that what is happening is actually explaining or discussing or even persuading. After all, the intent is to explain and convince. But in situations of conflict the difference between an explanation and a sermon tend to disappear very fast. This happens because the person on the other side is not actually open to "learning lessons" or being "shown the truth" in this way. This causes the explainer to feel frustrated, and to elevate the tenor of his or her "explanation" until the point is made. The tone becomes more emphatic and insistent, and what may have started out as an explanation soon turns into an all-out lecture. The spouse's reaction will be similar. The tougher the sermon, the stronger the rejection.

Coaching parents in relinquishing the drive to convince, which causes harsher and harsher arguments, is imperative for avoiding escalation. Relinquishing the drive to persuade does not mean relinquishing the goal. On the contrary, a unilateral act, made with recognition of the other's right to think and believe differently, has the best chance of advancing the goal.

Act with Total Transparency

Acting behind the other parent's back increases hostility and widens the rift between parents, thereby weakening both. The therapist should be very clear that this is not an option at all. By agreeing to a pact of secrecy or encouraging the parent in treatment to hide actions from the other spouse, therapists are adding to an unhealthy relationship, which they will soon leave worse off than when they entered the picture.

It is important that the parent taking unilateral steps do so with maximum transparency and openness, and report both in advance and subsequently on all the steps taken. A reliable and nonhostile report is an important tool for avoiding escalation. On the other hand, secrecy will increase hostility by creating a sense of suspicion, subterfuge, and deceit. The report keeps the rift between the parents from growing, even when the other parent shows no signs of interest. The report can be made in oral or written form, or could be presented indirectly via a mediator when communication has come to a complete standstill. It is also important to differentiate between information and criticism, and for the report to be free of blame. Below is an example of a communication delivered by a mother to a father who blamed her for all their son's problems and refused to come to counseling. Because communication between the parents was meager at best, the message was delivered to the father both orally and in writing:

When One Parent Refuses to Be Part of the Treatment

Dear Norman,

I would like to share with you the steps I am planning to take regarding Uri's problem. I am currently in counseling for parents with children with anxiety problems. This is the counseling I asked your brother to tell you about. I have already been to two meetings, and have realized that I need to stop giving in to Uri's demands and to clearly and efficiently define healthier boundaries separating him and me. I am going to get support in my efforts from a number of people. I have already spoken to your brother and his wife, and they are both willing to help. I will get support also from my two sisters, and two friends (Clara and Bennie). With their help I plan to make it clear to Uri that I will not perform a lot of the unreasonable services he has been demanding anymore. I will stop delivering food to his room, and won't cook according to his special demands any longer. I will also stop constantly chauffeuring him around to his activities and friends. I will have support from family and friends also when facing the tantrums I expect from Uri. I share every detail of my problem with Uri with my supporters. One of the things I learned in counseling is that blaming you or myself for Uri's problems doesn't help. There's also no point in sitting idly by and waiting for some solution to appear on its own. I understand that right now you are not ready to participate in my plan, and I respect your decision, especially in light of the fact that over the years I myself have been acting in a totally opposite way to the way I intend to act now. I plan to announce to Uri this week how I am going to act from now on, and the steps I am planning to take. I will give you a copy of the announcement, to keep you in the picture. Even if you continue having your doubts, I will keep you posted on everything that develops. I will be glad if later on you decide to join the process, whether through cooperation with me, or in your own way.

Sonya

Use Intermediaries to Deliver Messages

The use of mediators is one reliable method of reducing escalation between parents when only one is actively engaged in the therapeutic process. Experience in various types of conflict has shown that even the exact same messages, when delivered by an intermediary, arouse less resistance than when they are delivered directly. Parents of teenagers are usually well aware of this phenomenon. The very same suggestions, which the teen resisted forcefully when they were made by his parents, are accepted without difficulty when coming from a third person. The restraining influence of intermediaries stems from a number of factors. Intermediaries generally provoke less anger and irritation, in the eyes of the recipient, than the person we are in conflict with. They do not come "tainted" by the negative views that have become associated with the direct adversary, and therefore their suggestions are also free of prejudicial associations. There is no sense of defeat in accepting a suggestion made by a mediator, as there is in accepting one made by a rival. Also, bringing intermediaries into the picture adds a dimension of publicity to the interaction, which makes it harder for many individuals to resist outright what seem like reasonable suggestions and lowers the willingness to create a scene. The moderating influence of a third person can help parents who are in conflict, as long as the mediator is acceptable to both sides. Although therapists can, in some cases, act as the intermediary between the parents, frequently they will be too closely associated with the parent in treatment to be viewed as a true go-between. Involving an outside agent can be extremely difficult for many parents. Nevertheless, in situations of escalation and polarization, when communication is unattainable directly, it is worth making the effort and helping parents to overcome the inhibition around involving others in their difficult relationship. Sometimes even a small improvement in the parents' cooperation can bring about a vast improvement in the atmosphere at home. In other cases we have treated, a parent who at first refused to come for counseling later came, following a message delivered by an intermediary. In some cases they also made crucial contributions to the parents' success at coping with the anxiety.

Increase Involvement

In encouraging parents to act unilaterally, the therapist can help them to increase their own involvement. There are many ways in which this can be done: by investing time and effort; by planning and executing new steps; by breaking old habits; by enlisting support; or by clearly and efficiently delivering messages to the child. In all these ways parents stop being people irrelevant to the child's coping and increase their influence in leading the home life in new directions. A parent who acts alone can actually become an agent of change for the entire family. This change, though, can threaten the status of the other parent. So, for example, when a father, who thus far has been only marginally involved in the child's daily routines, increases his involvement with his son, the mother might feel that he is invading her territory. In such cases it is helpful for parents acting on their own to accompany the steps they take with clear expressions of respect for the role of the other parent. These messages, too, can be delivered either directly, or through a mediator. By encouraging parents to send such messages the therapist helps to ensure that the result of the actions will be to deepen their involvement with their child, but also to minimize resentment of the other parent. The willingness to state openly and directly that the increased involvement does not represent an encroachment on the other parent's importance or position helps to reduce suspicion and resistance.

A parent who is striving for change and is faced by resistance from a spouse might be driven to ask: "What good will all my hard work do if my spouse keeps on doing everything the old way?" The therapist can remind the parent of the idea of multiple inner voices we discussed earlier. Within the anxious child coexist voices advocating avoidance, and voices clamoring to cope. The positive voices might be weak, or unheard, but under the right conditions they can grow stronger and more vocal. The unilateral steps made by the active parent create fertile ground for this process, as long as the one-sided move is not accompanied by increased escalation and opposition between the parents.

A WORD ON SIBLINGS

An often overlooked fact about parents of anxious children is that they are rarely *only* the parents of anxious children. Most parents of a child with an anxiety disorder will also be the parents of at least one other child, who may suffer from anxiety as well, or may be quite different and less prone to anxiety. The effect of a child's anxiety on the personal boundaries in the home is not limited to the boundaries between child and parents, but can also significantly impact the interactions between siblings and the relationship of the parents to the sibling children.

Many parents express feelings of guilt over the differences in their relationship with the anxious child and the other children. Sometimes the guilt is toward the anxious child because of negative interactions, distress the child experiences, or resentment over the impact the anxiety has on them. Other times parents may feel critical toward themselves because of the need to devote more attention, time, or resources to the anxious child. They may feel the other children are being neglected or less attended to. There are no real rules for dealing with these complex systems and emotions. However, a number of strategies and principles together constitute useful guidelines for navigating these tricky waters.

It's Okay to Pay a Price—If You're Buying Something Valuable

The therapist can use this idea to help parents decide when the prices that are being paid by siblings are reasonable and justified. The principle is that, although children have different needs that will change over time, such that each child might at some point need more resources than others, it is important to see if those resources are actually being put into something that will make things better. In Chapter 3 we looked in detail at the concept of *family accommodation* to a child's anxiety. Family accommodation refers to all the ways in which parents adjust their routines to assist the child in avoiding the anxiety. This will almost inevitably affect siblings as well. For instance, when parents decide not to invite over guests because one child is socially anxious, all the siblings are affected. However, this is a price that is actually not "buying" something valuable. In fact, family accommodation has been shown repeatedly to make a child's symptoms progressively worse rather than better (Lebowitz, Panza, Su, & Bloch, 2012; Storch et al., 2007). So in essence, the parents are asking the siblings to make a significant sacrifice—which will only make matters worse (and ensure the need for even more accommodation as a consequence). This sounds truly unfair.

By contrast, parents who need to allocate financial resources to a child's treatment, to spend time taking a child to therapy, or practicing exposures, or who need to make some concessions to allow for a gradual overcoming of the anxiety, might also place demands or limitations on siblings. However, these prices, although they may be large, will be part of a process that helps the child to overcome the problem. This is both a more worthy cause and one that is likely to make the situation for all siblings improve over time. In other words, the therapist can help the parents to differentiate between prices that are being paid to make things better and prices that are going toward actually making things worse!

Teasing

One problem that the therapist may be confronted with, either through parent report or directly from the anxious is child, is the issue of being teased by siblings because of the anxiety. The teasing can take many forms such as name calling (scaredy-cat; chicken; coward; baby; sissy, etc.); imitation of children's behavior when they are anxious; talking about the anxiety problem with others whom the child would rather not know; deliberately triggering the anxiety (e.g., popping balloons when a child is phobic of them; turning out the lights when a child fears the dark; coughing near a child with contamination fears); telling frightening stories or information; and many other forms of picking on the anxious child. This kind of abuse can only serve to heighten the anxiety and lower the child's already vulnerable self-esteem, and confidence. Additionally, it may lead the child to feel more alone and less supported. Both of these results will usually lower the child's willingness to engage in steps aimed at overcoming the anxiety.

Many children will not comprehend the impact of their teasing on their anxious sibling, and view it in the way they might if it were them being teased. Namely, as something that is of little importance or consequence. For the anxious child, however, the experience can be dramatically different. Children suffering from anxiety may feel trapped between their own inner distress and the hounding from environment, leading to much suffering. Additionally, children who look to their parents for protection from these kinds of behaviors, and sees them actually laughing or simply ineffective in stopping the behavior, will be less inclined to view them as allies to whom to turn for help in overcoming the anxiety. Not addressing the teasing parents may be lowering their own ability to act as effective supporters for the child.

The therapist should encourage the parents to act determinedly to stop the teasing. Often, simply explaining to the siblings what the child is experiencing is enough to put a stop to the problem. Other times more direct action will be necessary to stop it. In taking this kind of action the parents are teaching important lessons to both children. They learn that their parents are willing to act as leaders and intervene when something is wrong in the family; they also learn that the parents do not view the anxiety as a laughing or joking matter and this reflects the supportive stance of accepting the validity of the anxious child's experience. Finally, if the parents are even partially successful, children will learn that their parents are willing and able to help them with problems—a lesson that may apply to overcoming anxiety as well.

When teasing is happening at school with classmates rather than at home with siblings, the therapist should be willing to engage with the school to find solutions to the problem. Having an expert talk to the class about anxiety, for example, in a way that would allow the children to identify with the experience of being anxious, or encouraging teachers to step up and act more firmly to stop the teasing can be helpful. The therapist should encourage the parents to be as open as possible with the school team about the child's anxiety so that teachers and counselors understand the importance of stopping the teasing.

Imposed Accommodation and Siblings

In some cases children with severe anxiety will attempt to forcefully impose accommodation on parents, for example, by forcing them to act in certain ways or by instituting prohibitions against some actions (Lebowitz, Vitulano, Mataix-Cols, & Leckman, 2011; Lebowitz, Vitulano, & Omer, 2011). The same kinds of coercion can also be directed toward siblings. Brothers and sisters might be prohibited from touching certain things, sitting in some places, or even saying particular words. Or in other cases, they may be forced to provide anxious children with special services, such as accompanying them places because of a fear of being alone or participating in compulsive rituals. In some cases siblings will become the object of obsessive children's fears and they will attempt to impose strict rules of avoidance to minimize contact with the sibling.

In such cases it is actually the sibling who is in need of, and has the right to, protection by the parents. It is both unjust and unhealthy to allow a child to force siblings to participate in the anxiety disorder in this way, and the siblings will look to the parents for support and protection.

262

In addition, in our experience when parents do not express clear determination to prevent such behaviors, the relationship between the siblings is most jeopardized, as the siblings realize they must fight for themselves and tensions run high. Even when parents are not immediately successful at curbing the coercive behavior, knowing that the parents see the problem and recognize the injustice can be a tremendous source of support for the siblings.

REFERENCES

Bianchi, S. M. (2000). Maternal employment and time with children: Dramatic change or surprising continuity? *Demography, 37*, 401–414.

Coley, R. L., & Morris, J. E. (2002). Comparing father and mother reports of father involvement among low-income minority families. *Journal of Marriage and Family, 64*, 982–997.

Cummings, E. M., Ballard, M., El-Sheikh, M., & Lake, M. (1991). Resolution and children's responses to interadult anger. *Developmental Psychology, 27*, 462–470.

Dadds, M. R., & Powell, M. B. (1991). The relationship of interparental conflict and global marital adjustment to aggression, anxiety, and immaturity in aggressive and nonclinic children. *Journal of Abnormal Child Psychology, 19*, 553–567.

Davies, P. T., & Cummings, E. M. (1994). Marital conflict and child adjustment: An emotional security hypothesis. *Psychological Bulletin, 116*, 387–411.

Grych, J. H., & Fincham, F. D. (1990). Marital conflict and children's adjustment: A cognitive-contextual framework. *Psychological Bulletin, 108*, 267–290.

Guryan, J., Hurst, E., Kearney, M. S., & National Bureau of Economic Research. (2008). *Parental education and parental time with children.* Cambridge, MA: National Bureau of Economic Research.

Lebowitz, E. R., Panza, K. E., Su, J., & Bloch, M. H. (2012). Family accommodation in obsessive–compulsive disorder. *Expert Review of Neurotherapeutics, 12*, 229–238.

Lebowitz, E. R., Vitulano, L. A., Mataix-Cols, D., & Leckman, J. (2011). Editorial perspective: When OCD takes over . . . The family! Coercive and disruptive behaviours in paediatric obsessive compulsive disorder. *Journal of Child Psychology and Psychiatry, 52,* 1249–1250.

Lebowitz, E. R., Vitulano, L. A., & Omer, H. (2011). Coercive and disruptive behaviors in pediatric obsessive compulsive disorder: A qualitative analysis. *Psychiatry, 74,* 362–371.

Manassis, K., & Hood, J. (1998). Individual and familial predictors of impairment in childhood anxiety disorders. *Journal of the American Academy of Child & Adolescent Psychiatry, 37,* 428–434.

Messer, S. C., & Beidel, D. C. (1994). Psychosocial correlates of childhood anxiety disorders. *Journal of the American Academy of Child & Adolescent Psychiatry, 33,* 975–983.

Storch, E. A., Geffken, G. R., Merlo, L. J., Jacob, M. L., Murphy, T. K., Goodman, W. K., . . . Grabill, K. (2007). Family accommodation in pediatric obsessive-compulsive disorder. *Journal of Clinical Child and Adolescent Psychology, 36,* 207–216.

Ancillary Issues

PART FOUR

Ancillary Issues

CHAPTER FOURTEEN

School Refusal and School Phobia

School refusal is a common problem and is often associated with childhood anxiety disorders. Parents feel helpless in the face of a child's refusal to attend school. Therapists can help return a child to school and restore the parents' sense of efficacy.

Key points in this chapter:

- The prevalence of school refusal.
- The relation between school refusal and anxiety.
- Tools for overcoming school refusal and school phobia.

School refusal is one of the most distressing problems encountered by parents of children suffering from anxiety. When a child refuses to go to school parents find themselves under tremendous pressure. They are expected by teachers, friends, each other, and themselves to be able to get the child to school. Not being able to do so poses a daily challenge to their authority, their parenting skills, and their self-esteem. The sense of helplessness experienced when a parent, rushing to get siblings organized, lunches packed, and themselves to work, is faced with a flat refusal to move is overpowering. School attendance is the single largest point of interaction between the adult as parent and society at large. Parents have almost complete independence in deciding how to raise their children. They can teach them any system of belief, live where they like, feed them the diet of their choice (within broad boundaries), and choose what they are to wear, but they are required by law to ensure their child's education. However, the rules of society that require parents to get their kid to school do not also provide them with the tools to do so; tools that are often all too necessary. The critical glares of those who hold a parent in contempt for not being able to ensure their child's attendance belie the fact that, faced with the same refusal, they would be equally helpless.

When children are very young, perhaps at the preschool age, it is a relatively simple matter to ensure that they attend school. Parents "merely" have to be determined enough to ignore their pleas or to physically lift children in and out of the car and into the school. But fast-forward the scene 10 short years and there are no longer simple answers for how to respond to school-refusing children. Attempting to physically force the child to go now seems less like a grown-up imposing a rule on a small child, and more like two individuals fighting. When this is the case we strongly recommend *not using physical force at all.* On the other hand, the parent may justly feel as though there are not many replacements to the tools that have been removed from the toolbox. The ability to physically take a child to school has not been replaced by a more age-appropriate substitute for the older child or adolescent who obstinately declines to attend.

Various causes can lead to school refusal, and anxiety disorders are among the most common of all. We briefly review in this chapter some of what is known about absenteeism and present a plan for dealing with school phobia and school refusal. The steps described in this chapter, like the SPACE Program described in detail in previous chapters, is aimed at parent implementation and is most suitable for situations in which the child is not actively engaged in overcoming the problem. When a child *is* working actively with a therapist to overcome school phobia the clinician should be guiding the process and the pace should be set in cooperation with the child (but note: Working actively means more than merely attending weekly sessions). However, many children with school refusal will have backed themselves into a metaphorical corner, unable to ask for help and choosing every morning to "wait out" the necessary time until it is too late to go or until parents must leave for work. In this situation the child may be too apprehensive to work cooperatively with a therapist and parents may find that the onus to take action rests entirely with them.

School Refusal

Absenteeism, or children's absences from school, is a serious concern for a large number of children in most developed countries, including the United States (Kearney, 2008). According to the National Center for Education Statistics' (United States Department of Education, Institute of Education Sciences, 2012) most recent report on the state of education:

> In 2011, when asked about their school attendance in the previous month, [only] 51 percent of 4th-grade students and 45 percent of 8th-grade students reported having perfect attendance. In that same year, 30 percent of 4th-grade students reported missing 1–2 days; 12 percent missed 3–4 days, and 7 percent missed 5 or more days of school in the previous month. Thirty-five percent of 8th-grade students missed 1–2 days, 13 percent missed 3–4 days, and 6 percent reported missing 5 or more days of school.

Many factors contribute to the likelihood of a child missing school, including excusable and inexcusable absences. Physical illness, serious and not, account for many missed days, as do parent-related factors and decisions. However, psychological and psychiatric conditions are among the most frequent causes of school refusal in otherwise healthy children. In systematic studies of school refusal (Egger, Costello, & Angold, 2003; Kearney & Albano, 2004), anxiety was found to be a major factor contributing to the problem and was associated with various fears. Anxiety was also related to a host of somatic complaints that led to missed school days such as headache, stomachache, and sleep problems.

For some children who refuse to attend school, or attempt to do so, turning each morning into an ordeal for parent and child, the fear might relate to a separation anxiety disorder. Going to school entails what is often the longest separation a child will have to face from parents or caregivers. For children who worry about their parents disappearing, getting into a car accident, or about other possible calamities, the extended separation can be an extreme challenge. For other children, going to school can trigger anxiety of a social nature. School is the place where children have to face other children, interact with them, and be judged by them. Many parents can recollect the trials they faced themselves as pupils. Performance fears can be triggered by the possibility of being called on by the teacher in class, having to give an oral presentation, or the need to participate in a sports event or activity. Even something as ordinary as recess can be a nightmare for children who are overcome by shyness when they have to speak to other children. And as many of the children we meet can attest, the school environment can be a "real jungle"—in which the strong and popular children are often deliberately or unwittingly cruel. Physical characteristics such as being overweight, wearing glasses or braces, being too short or to tall, too physically developed or not developed enough in comparison to peers, can all be the trigger for social aggression that can trigger anxiety and avoidance. Victims of such bullying, or other forms of school violence, are significantly more likely to be absent from school than other children (Dake, Price, & Telljohann, 2003).

Other fears can also contribute to a child's aversion to school. A child with a fear of contamination might perceive school as a hotbed of disease, germs, lice, or dirt. Once one starts looking for them, the signs of contamination and infection are unavoidable in an environment populated by hundreds of active children. The runny nose of a classmate, which most children will never consciously register in awareness, can seem like a flashing red warning sign to one who is overly vigilant about sickness and disease. Even a child who does not have a specific fear of contamination might be worried about becoming sick in school or having to throw up in front of other children, and the humiliation that this might engender. In other cases, generalized anxiety or perfectionism can mean that avoiding school is easier than trying to do everything just so, to get everything perfect. We have known many children who are easily bright and talented enough to do very well in school but are consistently being frustrated by their own need for perfection. Crossing out what you wrote in your notebook because the letters didn't seem to be perfectly shaped, for example, can quickly lead to ending up in trouble because you didn't get the homework written down in time.

When a child is coping with a learning disability or an attention deficit disorder, every day can be a huge challenge. Rather than an opportunity to gain praise and positive feedback, a learning problem can make school a series of trials that present children with the lesson that they are not up to par. Even with the growing knowledge and resources available to children with these difficulties, having to contend with the demands of the classroom can be infinitely frustrating. When a teacher is not well informed or when children have not been properly diagnosed, the problem is often compounded, as they are viewed as less intelligent or more lazy than their peers. In speaking to a group of parents recently I tried to emphasize this point in the following way:

We all recognize that different people are best suited for different jobs. The idea that everyone should have the same occupation, the same job, seems ludicrous. I love my job as a psychologist, but I know plenty of people who would rather do almost anything than have my job. And I can think of lots of careers that I would never want to have, though others swear they're the best job in the world. We're all different and everyone knows it—**when thinking about adults.** Now think about kids. Until they are about 18 they are all pretty much expected to have the same job. We call it school. Every child has to go to school and do just about the same thing: sit still on a chair for many hours each day learning the same things. Of course, there are different lessons, but most of them rely on the same small set of skills. Is it likely that something so drastic in human nature changes when we reach the age of 17 or 18? Does all the human diversity suddenly appear at that age? Of course not! Children are just as different from each other as adults. Of course, we want every child to get an education and perhaps it is unavoidable that they engage in similar tasks, but we need to recognize the fact that school presents some children with an impossible proposition. They get very little choice in the matter. They don't pick what they're learning, who is teaching or even who they will sit next to for endless hours. If they like it and they're good at it, it's great. If they don't, they have a real problem.

Going to school when you have a learning disability can be like being stuck in a job that you're not good at, but are not allowed to quit. Every day it's like coming to work and being greeted by a boss who frowns at you and lets you know that "You're the worst worker here but I'm not allowed to fire you; so sit down and do your job—badly." And then, at the

271

end of the day, getting told: "Well, you did poorly again—see you tomorrow!"

This description is rather bleak, and for many children school will be a place that fosters development, health, and to some extent even individuality. But for the child who experiences school in the way we describe it, it is easy to see why school refusal seems like the only response. It often seems that there are three main "hooks" that can pull children toward school and make it a place they would like to be. One of these is academics, and children who do well academically are more likely to continue to regularly attend. Another hook is that of social interaction. Even if children are not star pupils, they enjoy seeing their friends and are welcomed or admired by them, so school can be an inviting place. The third hook that many children experience is that of athletics. Children who excel at sports are often perceived as more socially skilled than they actually are by other children. Allowances are made for the star hitter or the best quarterback that are not made for the child who is clumsy or slow. However, if none of these three hooks are pulling a child effectively toward school, going each day can be daunting.

The Cycle of School Avoidance
Avoidance is the natural response to anxiety and will almost inevitably lead to more anxiety, and more avoidance. This pattern—of avoidance leading to more anxiety and more avoidance—holds across almost all anxiety disorders. When children suffering from a phobia avoid engaging in a situation that could mean confronting the feared stimulus, they forfeit the opportunities they might otherwise have to learn that the thing they are avoiding is not dangerous, or that they are capable of withstanding the anxiety. When this happens the anxiety will tend to get worse, making the possibility of overcoming the problem seem increasingly remote. The cycle is all the more powerful in the case of school phobia. A child who becomes fearful of going to school, for any of the reasons described earlier or others, and stays home from school, will almost always become more fearful, and more vehemently opposed to going to school. A number of factors contribute to this pattern.

First, the child learns that staying home is a real possibility. Many children "try" to refuse school but have little hope that they will actually be able to avoid going. A little bit like office complainers who grumble about their duties or threaten not to get them done but know they really have little choice, many children will voice their indignation about going to school, despite being inwardly resigned to the idea that school is inevitable. However, when a child is able to actually not go, refusal suddenly becomes a real possibility rather than a fantasy. School has now gone from an inevitable fact of life to a burden that can be avoided with sufficient determination or the right set of actions. Every child will miss some days of school, if even because of ordinary reasons like having the flu. But while being sick is only going to be an occasional occurrence, anxiety can recur with regularity on a daily basis.

When a child misses more than the occasional day of school another factor comes into play. After a few days of being out of school, many children will begin to fear the need to explain their absence to teachers or peers. Children who avoided school because of social anxiety will rapidly become worried about the questions their classmates might ask if they were to return. For many children this will serve to exacerbate the preexisting anxiety and heighten the need to stay home. Even the innocent questions of friendly or concerned peers can seem devastating in the mind of a shy child who is embarrassed about having had to stay home, and can drive further avoidance and more anxiety in a potentially endless cycle. The potential longevity of this cycle is exemplified by the fact that school refusal is a significant variable in predicting whether separation anxiety will be limited to childhood or persist into adulthood. Adults suffering from separation anxiety have been found to be more likely to have a history of school refusal as children (Silove, Manicavasagar, & Drobny, 2002).

Effects on General Functioning and Self-Esteem
As a child misses more and more school days, the effects on overall well-being, self-esteem, and general level of functioning accumulate. All children know that every healthy child goes to school. By extension, a child who is not regularly in school is unhealthy. Missing school will generally cause a child to see themselves as "sick," or otherwise different. Many children, as time passes, will begin to adopt this self-view more and more broadly, assuming the role of the unhealthy child. Compounded by the desire to avoid additional situations in which their

absenteeism would be discussed or require explanation, children may begin to avoid a broader range of social activities. In this way Boy Scouts, team sports, and other extracurricular activities are forgone. Many children will find putative replacements for these activities. Many will prefer the safety of online role-playing games or other computer-based activities to real-life endeavors.

Computer games offer what, to many children, seem like the perfect substitute to many normal activities. They are engaging and stimulating enough to ensure that the child is not bored; they are competitive and challenging so children gain a sense of accomplishment that replaces the accomplishments they would otherwise be focused on; and many of them are social enough in nature to prevent a sense of loneliness that without them might grow from continued self-isolation. Computer games can also be addictive in nature, rapidly expanding to fill the time that is being freed up by not engaging in other things. Computer games also have another advantage in the eyes of many school-avoiding children. They can be played at night.

Often the prolonged school refusal will be characterized by a reversal of the diurnal cycle. Children may take to being awake at night and sleeping late into the day. During the day they are confronted by frustrated parents and by the reminders of all the things they are no longer doing. At night they will generally have the house to themselves as parents and siblings sleep. In extreme cases children or adolescents may take to not leaving their room at all during the day, preferring to sleep as much as possible, and only come out at night when they will not be forced to confront the family or other visitors.

The effects of all these patterns on a child's self-esteem are typically negative. Viewing themselves as different, forgoing formerly pleasurable activities, facing criticism and disappointment from parents, and retreating into isolation all serve to create a negative self-view that only minimizes the likelihood of overcoming the problem. These are among the challenges faced by therapists and parents in cases of protracted school refusal.

TREATMENT

Most of the treatment for school-phobic children has focused on treating the symptoms of anxiety that are associated with school phobia. This is done either through psychopharmacological agents such as selective serotonin reuptake inhibitors (SSRI) (see Chapter 16 for a discussion of medication in childhood anxiety) or behavioral interventions such as cognitive behavioral therapy. There has been some evidence for the efficacy of treatment in mitigating the anxiety and reducing absenteeism (Bernstein et al., 2000; Heyne, Sauter, Van Widenfelt, Vermeiren, & Westenberg, 2011; King et al., 1998).

Generally, the principles and techniques of behavioral therapy described elsewhere in this book apply equally to a child who, because of anxiety, refuses to attend school. Gradual desensitization can be used by having the child practice being in or near the school for gradually increased lengths of time. Sometimes a first step will be to approach the gate of the school after hours and remain there for a short while until the anxiety subsides. As children begin to actually attend class, they might start by leaving after a single period and incrementally increase the length of time they remain in school. For many children, the knowledge that they can leave after a short time will alleviate the anxiety enough to enter school. Frequently, however, once they are in class they prefer to remain there rather than leave partway through the day. The attention drawn to them by leaving during the school day may be more aversive than actually staying in school until the day is over.

Cognitive restructuring can be used to address the anxious cognitions of a child relating to school and classroom attendance. Understanding the particular content of these thoughts for each specific child will be important in this regard. Children who think they will be sick in class can learn to question the probability of this actually happening or to ask themselves whether such an event would actually be as devastating and catastrophic as they have come to feel. Relaxation can be used to ease the entrance into school and to help a child refrain from leaving the classroom when feeling overwhelmed. One or two minutes of relaxing breathing will almost invariably spell the difference between bolting from the classroom or staying put.

However, for many children with school phobia and refusal, these skills and tools will be moot because the child will be too anxious to engage with a therapist and collaborate with treatment. A child who "successfully" refuses to go to school will find refusing to attend therapy an easy challenge; and parents who expend their energy on trying to get the child out the door in the morning may not have the energy to "go another round" in the afternoon. When a child is unwilling to work even gradually toward returning to school, parents find themselves between a rock and a hard place. School and society at large expect them to be getting the child to school in a regular fashion but they are helpless in the face of the child's stubborn refusal. The involvement of outside agents such as a truancy officer feels like a threat to their parental efficacy and to the child's future prospects, and this frightens most parents. This sense of threat from the outside can lead parents to provide excuses for the child's absences, thereby enabling the refusal and lowering the likelihood of the child agreeing to go.

The steps detailed below are not a perfect solution for this situation. There is, of course, no "one size fits all" for school phobia; the panacea is forever a fantasy rather than a reality. Some children will not return to normal functioning without a period of hospitalization and others will require additional supports to overcome the problem. However, by implementing these steps parents can escape the helplessness of having no tool to start addressing the problem. The therapist, working with the parents, can help guide them away from passive inefficacy and shift the dynamic toward a more proactive stance.

We emphasize that any one of these steps by itself is unlikely to be particularly helpful and stress the importance of consistently implementing all of them in concert. This allows for the creation of sufficient momentum, which can drive change in an otherwise intractable situation. By cherry picking those steps that seem most appealing, the overall efficacy is significantly reduced.

Set Specific Expectations

The level of school attendance expected from the child will vary from case to case and will change as the process continues. For some children the initial level of expectation might be that they attend the first lesson of each day. In other cases it will be complete and full school attendance. In other cases it might be no more than getting in the car and driving to school without ever getting out of the car. The level of expectation should be set by therapist and parents, with the child's input when possible. Factors that will impact the expectation will include the level of attendance that has been occurring previously, the length of time since the child attended regularly, the level of anxiety reported and manifested by the child, and any other relevant variables.

Stop Unhelpful Talk

Do not talk about school or attendance. The absolute maximum discussion of the topic should be saying *once* each day: "You need to go to school tomorrow," or a comparable statement reflecting the level of expectation that has been determined. Apart from the single iteration of that expectation, the only other school refusal–related talk is in the morning, when the parents wake the child. When they are awake parents should say one time: "It is time to go to school—you need to go now." If the child refuses to go, the discussion ends immediately.

Repeatedly discussing the issue of school without actual change occurring strengthens the parents' sense of helplessness and highlights their inability to be effective, in the eyes of the child. If the parents have in the past engaged in endless conversations, lectures, pleading, or threats about the topic of school and all to no avail, then one more such conversation is unlikely to make the difference and will actually serve to weaken their stance. Most of the time children will have long since become inured to this kind of talk and see it as the relatively small price they must pay for continuing their absence from the classroom. Some parents (and some therapists) might find the notion of *not* discussing the school attendance counterintuitive or even paradoxical. It can be explained in the following way:

> Imagine that you are a manager in a place of work and that you have an employee who arrives late for work one day. You might call him into your office, explain that this is a business and that he needs to be on time. Imagine that your employee nods understandingly and the next morning arrives late again. You would call him back into your office again and reiterate that he absolutely must arrive to work on time. He might nod his head, agree with you and the next morning . . . arrive late again. Say that this pattern went on for some months. If, after some months you are still repeating the same words every morning, then consider what message you are sending. Is your worker hearing 'You need to be at work on time' or do you actually seem to be saying 'I want you to be at work on time but

am completely at a loss about how to make sure you do that'. Is this the message you want to be sending to a child about school attendance? Before you can act effectively you need to stop reinforcing the message that there is nothing effective for you to do!

Maintain Connections with Peers and Teachers

One of the things that makes school refusal appealing for many anxious children is the possibility of avoiding contact with classmates and teachers. Generally, if children are "successful" at not going to school this will mean that they will not have to contend with seeing any school-related people for another day. We recommend dissolving this equation. Invite children to come visit the child at home. Ask teachers to call or stop by the home as frequently as possible. By creating a regular stream of "school people" in the home, the benefit of not going to school is very much reduced. In fact, within a short period of time it may seem like not going actually increases the need to deal with peers and staff.

Make sure that the child knows what schoolwork is being done, what homework assignments are given, and about all other school-related activities and events. Maintaining a constant connection with school life will mitigate the effect that absenteeism can have on a child's sense of identity. Rather than seeing themselves as detached from school life they can continue to perceive themselves as students. This effect can be magnified by classmates' visits to the home. In one case classmates photographed an absent child's empty chair and brought her the picture saying: "See, your place is waiting for you. We want you back!"

Invite Classmates to Accompany the Child to School in the Morning

This is one of the most effective tools for combating school refusal. It does, however, require some coordination with teachers and parents of classmates. Ask the teacher for collaboration. In the best cases teachers have been very much on board and have created a rotation of children who would stop by the school-refusing child's home on the way to school to invite them to go with them. Ask the parents to call the parents of other children they know and ask for their help. Most parents will be agreeable if their child does not object. Have them offer to pick up classmates in the morning from home and to bring them to school even if the child does not agree to go. Even if the child refusing school objects to these "invasions" into the home, the rule should explicitly be that as long as they are not going to school independently there is no choice but to do everything possible to help them.

Ask for the Help of Friends, Family, and Primary Care Practitioners

Make a list of family members, friends, colleagues, and others and ask them to contact the child and emphasize the need to go to school. There is no need for lecturing or criticism. Ask them to say simply: "I've heard you've been having trouble getting to school recently. I understand that can be hard. You should know that it is your absolute obligation to go to school and your parents are required by law to send you." The message can be given in person, by phone, by letter, or in any other way.

Minimize the Temptations of Staying Home

Identify the pleasurable aspects of staying home and try to minimize them. If children are playing computer games for most of the day, disconnect the computer. If they are on the phone, remove phone privileges. If they are ordering pizza or fast food for lunch, prepare a school lunch and leave it for them. If they are spending the time talking to parents or siblings, try to impose a "you're in school" rule where contact is limited to after school hours only. Children who are faced with the choice between going to school after a prolonged absence and spending hours playing their favorite game are unlikely to choose the former. Do not help the child to escape feeling bored. Although it is true that children should not be punished for being anxious, the removal of these activities is not a punishment. It is a tool to enable them to get better.

REFERENCES

Bernstein, G. A., Borchardt, C. M., Perwien, A. R., Crosby, R. D., Kushner, M. G., Thuras, P. D., & Last, C. G. (2000). Imipramine plus cognitive-behavioral therapy in the treatment of school refusal. [Clinical Trial Comparative Study Randomized Controlled Trial Research Support, Non-U.S. Gov't Research Support, U.S. Gov't,

P.H.S.]. *Journal of the American Academy of Child & Adolescent Psychiatry,* 39(3), 276–283.

Dake, J. A., Price, J. H., & Telljohann, S. K. (2003). The nature and extent of bullying at school. [Review]. *Journal of School Health, 73*(5), 173–180.

Egger, H. L., Costello, E. J., & Angold, A. (2003). School refusal and psychiatric disorders: A community study. [Research Support, Non-U.S. Gov't Research Support, U.S. Gov't, P.H.S.]. *Journal of the American Academy of Child & Adolescent Psychiatry, 42*(7), 797–807.

Heyne, D., Sauter, F. M., Van Widenfelt, B. M., Vermeiren, R., & Westenberg, P. M. (2011). School refusal and anxiety in adolescence: Non-randomized trial of a developmentally sensitive cognitive behavioral therapy. [Clinical Trial]. *Journal of Anxiety Disorders, 25*(7), 870–878.

Kearney, C. A. (2008). School absenteeism and school refusal behavior in youth: A contemporary review. [Comparative Study Review]. *Clinical Psychology Review, 28*(3), 451–471.

Kearney, C. A., & Albano, A. M. (2004). The functional profiles of school refusal behavior. Diagnostic aspects. [Comparative Study]. *Behavior Modification, 28*(1), 147–161.

King, N. J., Tonge, B. J., Heyne, D., Pritchard, M., Rollings, S., Young, D., . . . Ollendick, T. H. (1998). Cognitive-behavioral treatment of school-refusing children: A controlled evaluation. *Journal of the American Academy of Child & Adolescent Psychiatry, 37*(4), 395–403.

Silove, D., Manicavasagar, V., & Drobny, J. (2002). Associations between juvenile and adult forms of separation anxiety disorder: A study of adult volunteers with histories of school refusal. *Journal of Nervous and Mental Disease, 190*(6), 413–415.

United States Department of Education, Institute of Education Sciences. (2012). *The condition of education.* Washington, DC: National Center for Education Statistics.

CHAPTER FIFTEEN

Highly Dependent Young Adults

Anxiety disorders are one cause of the rising prevalence of highly dependent adult children who are living with their parents and unable to function independently as mature individuals. In these cases parents and children are caught in a trap of dependency and mutual frustration. In this chapter we discuss the phenomenon and present two cases that illustrate the scenario and avenues for change.

Key points in this chapter:

- The growing prevalence of highly dependent adult children.
- The role of parent training in addressing the situation.

Low-functioning grown children who are highly dependent on their parents are a growing phenomenon in many parts of the world. This trend is reflected in the coining of many special words to describe the situation: In Japan they are called *Hikikomori* (Malagon, 2010), in Italy *Bamboccioni*, in Germany and France *Tanguy Syndrome* (Janne, 2007), and in England (Finlay, Sheridan, McKay, & Nudzor, 2010) *NEET* (not in employment, education, or training) or *Kippers* (kids in parents' pockets eroding retirement savings). In Canada they are termed *Boomerang Children* (Ravanera, Rajulton, & Burch, 1995; Settersten, Furstenberg, & Rumbaut, 2005), in

Austria *Mamma's Hotel Children*, and in South Korea they are known as *Kangurus*.

In the United States the phenomenon has been given various names including the "Full Nest Syndrome" (Schnaiberg & Goldenberg, 1989; White, 1994) and "ILYA" (incompletely launched young adult). The phenomenon was also brought to popular attention under the name *Failure to Launch*, in a movie by the same name in which parents hired a relationship expert to help lure their 35-year-old son away from their all-too-comfortable home and toward independence.

In Greece, Italy, Portugal, and Spain, well over half of all young adults currently live with their parents (Giuliano, 2007). In the United Kingdom and North America rates are significantly higher compared to past decades (Berrington, Stone, & Falkingham, 2009; Settersten et al., 2005), and in Japan there are estimated to be millions of self-isolating and dependent adults who have aroused considerable social and financial concern (Teo, 2010).

Temporarily living at home and receiving help from one's parents may be a normative phase that allows young people to find their way in life. In many cases, however, the transition to fully autonomous functioning does not occur or is reversed after an abortive attempt at independence (Goldscheider & Goldscheider, 1998, 1999), leading to chronic dependence on parental support. Research has indicated the presence of significant populations of chronically dysfunctional young adults with various diagnostic labels who pose considerable burden to themselves and society (Pepper, Kirshner, & Ryglewicz, 2000).

Alongside individual and family characteristics, a number of socio-cultural factors may contribute to the spread of overly dependent grown children: (a) Modern society's prolongation of adolescence as a period of search for personal, professional, and social identity creates a situation in which it is less and less clear when the young person should be expected to function independently (Arnett, 2007); (b) the belief that all people should find a career that perfectly suits their personality sanctifies the right for a personal search that may at times become interminable (Collin & Young, 2000; Twenge, 2006); (c) the decrease in traditional parental authority makes parents less able to set demands and limits (Omer, 2011); and (d) the spread of computer technology presents people with the temptation of a virtual life that satisfies their needs for entertainment and occupation without exposing them to the wear and tear of the "real world" (Shaw & Black, 2008).

The affluence of the Western world may allow some families to sustain adults who do not work without experiencing excessive financial burden, but research has indicated that parents of higher socioeconomic status express greater levels of dissatisfaction with the situation, perhaps holding higher expectations for financial independent success (Aquilino, 1990). Although culture-specific factors presumably impact attitudes toward staying at home, it would appear from the data presented earlier that both collectivistic societies that emphasize strong family ties and individualistic ones that emphasize personal choice in career development may foster dependence in today's world.

Although the diagnostic characteristics of such individuals are varied, anxiety seems to play a major role in creating these situations. Social anxiety is often triggered by the need to face new challenges as an individual matures. The need to participate in job interviews, for example, can cause someone to recoil from the challenges of becoming self-supporting. Young adults with obsessive-compulsive disorder may feel overwhelmed by the need to independently create schedules and adhere to them, and those with generalized anxiety disorder may feel incapable of the kind of decision making that independent life or higher education require. For instance, some potential college students faced for the first time with the opportunity to independently choose a place to learn or curricula to focus on may become entrenched in doubt and unable to make any decisive choice. Panic disorder and agoraphobia can also severely impair the ability to function outside of the home. Although in some cases the pressures of adulthood can trigger anxiety or exacerbate less severe existing symptoms in others, the adult status is merely the continuation of a longer-term process of avoidance, impairment, or isolation. Although some parents look forward to adulthood as a time when their child will by necessity overcome anxiety and become more autonomous, this hope is often unfounded. The school-refusing or socially phobic child may simply grow into a very similar adult.

The Dependency Trap

In a related paper we described such individuals using the term *Adult Entitled Dependence* or AED (Lebowitz, Dolberger, Nortov, & Omer, 2012) and used the term *dependency trap* in an attempt to capture the kind of dynamic that we have often encountered in their families. The dependency trap describes a situation in which the family seems caught in a vicious cycle in which attempts by both the dependent individual and the parents to alleviate the condition actually exacerbate it.

The dependent adult may try to alleviate the distress she feels, for example, by pressing for ever more parental protection or services. However, the increased protection and accommodation can actually reduce her ability to cope independently. The parents, in turn, might feel obliged to come to their children's rescue, but the more they do so, the less they appear able to function on their own. Occasionally, frustration may lead parents to pose impulsive and rigid demands. The dependent adults respond in kind, escalating their behavior, perhaps even through an exhibit of violence or suicidality, after which the parents retreat into the more familiar accommodating style.

Among the families of dependent adult children whom we have studied (Lebowitz et al., 2012), parents usually were engaged in the provision of many services that appear inappropriate to the age and putative functional capacity of the child. For example, although many of the children were well into their twenties or thirties, parents were providing services such as laundry, shopping, cooking, and driving to various places. In most cases the adult children also were financially reliant on their parents and often demanded quite significant amounts of money (for example, for computers or Internet access) that the parents felt they had no choice but to provide. It is likely that the avoidance and consequent dependence of the grown child on the parent promote a more general dependent style that is broadly applied across many domains. Another unfortunate consequence of the dependency trap in many of the families we encountered was the prevalence of aggressive and even violent behavior on the part of the grown children when confronted with what they perceived as inadequate accommodation to their needs. Parents may fluctuate between at times seeing their child as weak, helpless, and desperately in need of their assistance and at other times wishing to promote more independence but fearing the negative consequences of defying the inappropriate demands.

Some of the work we have done in this field has been aimed at learning more about the kinds of accommodating behaviors that parents were engaged in, as well as probing the underlying beliefs that might be causing the parents to have more difficulty curtailing them. Earlier work had pointed to a fundamental conflict between parents' desire to protect their children and the wish to launch them into full and independent adulthood (Schnaiberg & Goldenberg, 1989). This echoes, in a kind of adult version, the conflicts we have described in earlier chapters that face parents of anxious children of younger ages. The perceived discrepancy between the parental protective role and the role of better preparing and equipping a child for life's challenges is pervasive among parents of anxious children. It also highlighted the possibility that the same principles that apply in guiding parents of younger anxious children would be applicable or translatable for adult-dependent children. The table below shows a list of some of the statements that parents of dependent adult children endorsed (Na'man, 2011). These included cognitions and ideas that parents held, descriptions of parental accommodating behaviors, and statements that reflected the negative consequences that the dependency trap was having on family life.

Statements endorsed by parents of adult highly dependent children
My child is overly dependent on me for his age and capabilities.
I supply my child with services in various domains that are beyond those expected for his age and capabilities.
I feel my child cannot make it in life without my help.
I mediate most of my child's contact with the "outside world" because of his avoidance.
I feel my personal life is significantly restricted because of the need to meet my child's needs and demands.
I make changes to my work routine because of the need to accommodate my child's needs and demands.

(Continued)

I do not engage in hobbies or relationships because of my child's objections.
My family and my household are negatively impacted by the need to accommodate my child's needs and demands.
I have assumed responsibilities or taken over tasks that my child should be in charge of.
I feel I have no choice but to provide these services to my child.
I allow my child to isolate in his room, though I know this is not good for him.
I meet my child's demands for services such as shopping, television, driving, or cooking favorite foods.
I am so used to providing these services that I can have difficulty imagining stopping.
I believe that if I do not take care of my child and provide services, his mental or physical health will deteriorate.
Because of my child's needs and demands the whole family is restricted.
I feel distress because of the need to meet my child's needs and demands.
I fear that if I act differently my child might respond with rage or violence.
In the past, attempts to accommodate less only made things worse.
I have a special sensitivity to my child's needs.
Sometimes I fill my child's needs without being asked.

The principles and tools described in earlier chapters and detailed in the SPACE Program offer parents a way of supporting an anxious child, decreasing accommodation, and improving functioning. The challenges of applying those principles to adult low functioning and highly dependent individuals are significant but surmountable. Among these

286

challenges are the longer amount of time that the child has often been avoidant or even self-isolating, leading to more entrenched behavioral patterns; the lesser degree of authority that parents typically have in regard to adult children as opposed to minors; the decrease in services and supports available to parents of adult children compared to child-hood or adolescent services; the fear of physical confrontation is often greater as is the perceived risk of suicidality (though this is not neces-sarily well founded).

Nevertheless, in a preliminary study (Lebowitz et al., 2012) involving the parents of 27 highly dependent adult children, parents were able to achieve significant change in parent training that applied similar tech-niques. The following case examples demonstrate both the immense challenges and complexity of addressing these situations and the potential for change in what may appear to be insurmountable cohesion. Little work has been done in characterizing or treating this kind of dependence in adults but there appears to be much needed for further research and development in this field.

Case I

Eli and Myra, the parents of George (18) and Gina (13), asked for help with George's self-isolation. They described him as an intelligent and sensitive person who had been a good student with an active social life, and with whom, until recently, they had shared a warm and close relationship. About a year before the beginning of treatment, George developed a deep aversion to Gina. He avoided staying in one room with her or touching any object that might have been touched by her. He would curse her and complain about her presence in the home. George's aversion gradually developed into a rigid set of rules that were imposed on the whole household. His clothes had to be laundered separately, the air-conditioning had to stay off because it might con-taminate the air in his room with Gina's breath, and he refused to eat any food that came out of the kitchen. He demanded a private refrigerator in his room and his mother had to bring him food from outside the house. He would only go out occasionally when his mother took him in her car, but she had to guarantee that Gina would never sit on the front seat that was reserved for him. George developed a similar aversion toward his father, blaming him for ruining his life. He called him "pedophile" but refused to say why. He would not leave his room unless Myra guaranteed that he would not see his father. George stopped going to school, severed all social ties, and inverted his diurnal cycle.

After many failed attempts to get in touch with his son, Eli became resigned. In the first session with the therapist he burst into tears, saying: "It's been six months since I last saw my son. I don't remember what he looks like!"

George rejected professional help, stating that the real problems were his father and sister. The parents in turn felt that nobody could help them and kept their situation a closely guarded secret.

The therapist explained to the parents that George was probably suffering from OCD. He added that accommodation to his demands, though stemming from love and compassion, exacerbated George's condition. He suggested the family begin to resist the "tyranny" of George's OCD over the family.

The parents were informed of the importance of having a network of supporters to help them in their struggle. Despite initial unwillingness to lift the veil of secrecy, Eli talked to his brothers and to a couple of friends and was surprised by their warm reaction. In the supporter meeting that took place a few weeks later, 17 people participated. Eli and Myra felt a surge of energy at the impressive commitment displayed by the group.

Nonetheless, as the details of the upcoming struggle became clearer, their initial optimism gave way to paralyzing fears. Myra was terrified that any challenge to the status quo might cause George to suffer a psychotic break or possibly even lead to his suicide. Eli feared that renewed friction between himself and George could lead to physical violence. It soon became clear that Myra was too apprehensive to act, so the focus shifted to enabling Eli to undertake the first steps unilaterally. Eli objected: "I will do nothing without Myra's agreement!" Myra smiled ironically and said: "And I will do nothing without George's agreement!" Myra's words had a provocative edge, which gave an opening to the therapist. He said: "I think Myra is aware of the absurdity of the situation and may be asking us to challenge it. She was being ironic when she said that she would do nothing without George's agreement. She has already said that she is overburdened with George's demands and would like nothing better than getting your help in dealing with the problem. I think she is now telling us that if you take the initiative, she will be able to cope with that!" Myra nodded approvingly. The therapist then added to Eli: "I think you should act to reclaim your fatherhood!" Eli reacted warmly.

The parents came to the following session with an astounding proposal: Myra would travel abroad for 10 days, leaving the field open for Eli's initiative. She offered not to participate in the sessions in which a plan of action was being prepared, so that her emotional reactions would not hinder the process. Eli came to the meetings with a brother and two cousins, who would be his immediate supporters in the operation. The plan was: Eli would enter George's room (by force if necessary) on the very day of Myra's flight abroad and stay there until the situation calmed down. He would unilaterally break the communication taboo, abolish the sterile rules that had been imposed on the house, and declare he would resist George's abuse against him and Gina. The three supporters would be in the house and help him in case of need.

When Eli entered the room, George protested loudly and tried to push him out. The supporters drew closer to prevent the situation from deteriorating into outright violence, whereupon George started yelling: "He's a pedophile!" All the supporters took turns staying in the room with George, sometimes with Eli and sometimes without. After two hours George was ready to talk. When he again called his father a pedophile his uncle told him: "If you say this again, I will call the police and you will be required to make a formal statement." By the end of the day George was talking to his father, without looking him in the face. He agreed to leave the house every day, to buy food for himself, and to allow Eli to enter the room when he knocked. Eli and the supporters were surprised to discover that George's refrigerator had been completely stocked by his mother before her trip. She had done this without telling Eli.

When Myra returned she followed Eli's example in resisting some of George's rules. She told him she no longer forbade Gina's sitting in the front seat. George protested, but did not boycott the car. After the parents showed him written documentation of his verbal abuse of Gina and stated that they would share the documentation with the supporters if it was repeated, the abuse ceased.

In the following weeks George started going out every day, met with friends, began taking driving lessons, and eventually passed his driving test. He still refused to look his father in the eyes or to initiate any conversation with him. However, he always answered and sometimes a short conversation developed.

Five months later George started his military service, finished basic training successfully, and was given a responsible job in the military working with computers.

Case II

Simon and Silvia described their son Ben (26) as delicate and conscientious. He lived at home, worked sporadically when opportunity presented itself, and studied inconsistently. He went to the gym a few times a week, but mostly stayed in his room, lying in bed or at the computer. Ben felt ashamed when meeting with friends who, in his eyes, had already achieved something in their lives. His parents gave him a car, hoping that this would encourage him to go out, but he used it only to go to the gym. On rare occasions, when the parents dared to make any demands, Ben reacted aggressively, which was doubly frightening because it seemed so out of character.

Simon would invite Ben to go to a restaurant with him once a week to keep the parent-son relationship alive. Ben came willingly but would block any attempt at personal or challenging conversation. If asked about his plans for the future, Ben would answer: "You will see, I will still surprise you all!" Or "I know that the right thing for me will come along!"

Ben's parents were terrified of doing anything that might disrupt the delicate fabric of their relationship with him. They feared that taking a firmer stance would lead to a deep rupture or further damage Ben's condition. They would have gladly sent Ben to individual therapy for as long as necessary, but he refused to even consider the option.

When the therapist broached the topic of practical steps that would need to be taken, such as delivering a written announcement, mobilizing supporters, or discontinuing Internet service, Silvia was horrified. Simon was highly skeptical of Ben's ability to function in a meaningful way: "What is waiting for him out there?" he asked, "Working as a waiter won't get him anywhere!" When asked how Ben would react to a determined action on the part of the parents Simon said: "He will withdraw completely for a very long time!"

Gradually the parents became convinced that only unilateral action could trigger a process of change. A supporters' meeting was convened with five members of the extended family. It was agreed that the parents would deliver an announcement to Ben stating they would no longer accept his staying at home without studying or going to work. They wrote that they would be willing to help rent an apartment for the first months. The supporters were to contact Ben and offer their help in dealing with the new situation. His uncle, with whom Ben had been close in the past, would invite him to his house for a couple of weeks.

When the parents told Ben they wanted to give him a written message, he warned them: "Don't do that! You will cause big damage!" The parents were undaunted and delivered the announcement. Ben took the letter to his room, came down screaming, took out a bundle of banknotes from his pocket, tore them to pieces and threw the bits in his father's face yelling: "You see! This is money that I earned, working. Now you have spoiled everything! Everything! Because of you I am not going to work again!" He then burst into tears and went back to his room.

Ben avoided all contact with his parents for days after their announcement. Simon would talk to Ben, but received no answer. He spoke quietly, but made it clear that the present situation could not continue. Ben did not repeat his tantrum, choosing instead to withdraw into himself, as his father had predicted.

It took more than 2 months before the parents were prepared to take another step. They told Ben they would disable the computer during the night and discontinue Internet access. This time Ben showed more positive signs of coping. He began leaving the house early in the morning (he was working—the parents soon found a paycheck on his table) and after a few weeks he came back with a laptop computer, which he was able to connect to the neighbors' wireless Internet network. He surprised his parents once again by leaving them a message that he was flying abroad with friends for 10 days. This was doubly surprising, because Ben had suffered from a fear of flying in the past! The parents were in high spirits. However, when Ben returned from his trip he reverted to the old pattern. He now had his own computer and Internet, with which he kept the world at bay.

It was now clear that Ben could withstand pressure without submitting to demands. The parents also understood it was vain to hope that the problem would be solved on Ben's own initiative. They told Ben they would no longer allow him to use the computer or watch TV in their house. If he did so, they would remove the computer from the house. They also told him they were renting him a small apartment. They would no longer agree to his living in their house without any occupation. Ben shut himself up in his room for a number of days, coming out only in the middle of the night to eat in the kitchen.

One morning the parents found a note on the door of their room that read: "Conditions for capitulation: You must write a letter to all the people you have involved, apologizing for your offending my honor. Also, you have to donate 3.000 NIS (about $800) to the Israel Democracy Institute as compensation for your tyrannical acts. When I see the letter and the receipt from the Institute I will agree to leave." At first the bewildered parents wanted to refuse the ultimatum. However, after discussing it with the therapist, they came to see it as Ben looking for a way of protecting his dignity and self-respect, accepting their demand without complete capitulation. They accepted the conditions and a few days later brought him the letter and receipt. They rented an apartment and after he procrastinated for a few days, Ben moved there.

Apart from rent, the parents stopped giving Ben money. After a few weeks it became clear that Ben was working. He was using the car to travel to friends far away and he paid for his own subscription to the gym. For months he did not talk to his parents, though he kept contact with them in a peculiar way. He would come to visit the house when the parents were at work and leave tell-tale signs of his presence. He would eat a little (a yogurt, an apple), but would leave the cooked food in the fridge untouched. He never took any food products from the house. Simon was in touch with two of Ben's friends, who told him that Ben went to pubs, visited them at their houses, and drove to visit other friends in other parts of the country.

Half a year after he had left the house, Ben met the parents at a family wedding. He sat at their table and conducted some small talk with them, without telling them anything about his doings. This happened again a month later. The parents started to leave messages for Ben on the kitchen table. They wrote that they respected Ben's decision to keep his doings private. They said they missed him a lot, but understood that things had to be done at his own pace. The parents were sad about the lack of contact, but satisfied with what they had achieved, feeling that Ben was now looking for ways to lead his life without isolation or dependence. In the first months they thought that Ben was punishing them by distancing himself from them. Gradually, however, they came to see that Ben was protecting himself from the emotional reactions he feared would overwhelm him should he get any closer to his parents.

REFERENCES

Aquilino, W. S. (1990). The likelihood of parent-adult child coresidence: Effects of family structure and parental characteristics. *Journal of Marriage and Family, 52*(2), 405–419.

Arnett, J. J. (2007). Emerging adulthood: What is it, and what is it good for? *Child Development Perspectives, 1*(2), 68–73.

Berrington, A., Stone, J., & Falkingham, J. (2009). The changing living arrangements of young adults in the UK. *Population Trends* (138), 27–37.

Collin, A., & Young, R. A. (2000). *The future of career.* New York, NY: Cambridge University Press.

Finlay, I., Sheridan, M., McKay, J., & Nudzor, H. (2010). Young people on the margins: In need of more choices and more chances in twenty-first century Scotland. *British Educational Research Journal, 36* (5), 851–867.

Giuliano, P. (2007). Living arrangements in Western Europe: Does cultural origin matter? *Journal of the European Economic Association, 5*(5), 927–952.

Goldscheider, F. K., & Goldscheider, C. (1998). The effects of childhood family structure on leaving and returning home. *Journal of Marriage and the Family, 60*(3), 745–756.

Goldscheider, F. K., & Goldscheider, C. (1999). *The changing transition to adulthood: Leaving and returning home.* Thousand Oaks, CA: Sage.

Janne, P. (2007). Revisiting the "Tanguy" phenomenon: About retarded self-sufficiency in our post-adolescent population. *Therapie familiale, 28*(2), 167–180.

Lebowitz, E. R., Dolberger, D., Nortov, E., & Omer, H. (2012). Parent training in non violent resistance for adult entitled dependence. *Family Process, 51*(1), 1–17.

Malagon, A. (2010). "Hikikomori": A new diagnosis or a syndrome associated with a psychiatric diagnosis? *International Journal of Social Psychiatry, 56*(5), 558–559.

Na'man, T. (2011). *Development and validation of the Parents Accommodation Scale (PAS) among parents of an adult child living at home.* (Master's thesis), Tel Aviv University, Tel Aviv.

Omer, H. (2011). *The new authority: Family, school, community.* New York, NY: Cambridge University Press.

Pepper, B., Kirshner, M. C., & Ryglewicz, H. (2000). The young adult chronic patient: Overview of a population. *Psychiatric Services, 51*(8), 989–995.

Ravanera, Z. R., Rajulton, F., & Burch, T. K. (1995). A cohort analysis of home-leaving in Canada, 1910–1975. *Journal of Comparative Family Studies, 26*(2), 179.

Schnaiberg, A., & Goldenberg, S. (1989). From empty nest to crowded nest: The dynamics of incompletely-launched young adults. *Social Problems, 36*, 251.

Settersten, R. A., Furstenberg, F. F., & Rumbaut, R. G. (2005). *On the frontier of adulthood: Theory, research, and public policy.* Chicago, IL: University of Chicago Press.

Shaw, M., & Black, D. W. (2008). Internet addiction: Definition, assessment, epidemiology and clinical management. *CNS Drugs, 22*(5), 353–365.

Teo, A. R. (2010). A new form of social withdrawal in Japan: A review of Hikikomori. *International Journal of Social Psychiatry, 56*(2), 175–185. doi:10.1177/0020764008100629

Twenge, J. M. (2006). *Generation me: Why today's young Americans are more confident, assertive, entitled—And more miserable than ever before.* New York, NY: Free Press.

White, L. (1994). Coresidence and leaving home—Young adults and their parents. *Annual Review of Sociology, 20*, 81–102.

CHAPTER SIXTEEN

Medication for Childhood Anxiety

Medication can be an effective way to treat childhood anxiety. The decision to use medication is complex and requires careful consideration. In this brief chapter we discuss the use of medication for the treatment of anxiety and present information on common medications.

Key points in this chapter:

- Medication can be effective in treating anxiety.
- Medication can be combined with cognitive behavioral therapy.
- Common medications for treating anxiety.

Keeping in mind that every human thought or emotion has a physiological counterpart in the brain, it comes as no surprise that it is possible to influence these functions through the use of medications that work on the nervous system. This is certainly true of anxiety and anxiety disorders. Anxiety is first and foremost a response of the nervous system, an alarm raised when threat is perceived. Psychopharmacological agents can have a dramatic effect on the way the alarm is sounded, on the reactions it evokes, and on the behavior that ensues.

Alongside evidence-based psychotherapeutic interventions such as cognitive behavioral therapy, the use of medication has revolutionized the treatment of childhood anxiety disorders in the past decades. A large body of evidence supports the usefulness of psychopharmacological agents in the treatment of children's anxiety. These two modalities, psychotherapy and medication, have been found to be helpful both when used individually and when the two are combined so that a child is treated with both CBT and medication. The combination can be either sequential or simultaneous. When the treatments are provided sequentially the order could either start with CBT and then introduce medication (as in cases where the improvement has been unsatisfactory) or start with medication and then begin psychotherapy (as in when the severity of symptoms or other factors preclude initiating therapy until some improvement is achieved).

The number of studies that have compared either treatment, provided individually, to the combination of both psychotherapy and medication is much smaller than the number of treatment studies that have investigated only one treatment modality. From the data accumulated so far the tentative conclusion is that the combination of CBT and medication is somewhat superior to either treatment on its own. For example, in a large study of treatment for childhood anxiety that compared the effect of CBT, medication (sertraline), or the combination of both, the combined treatment was significantly more effective than either treatment alone (Walkup et al., 2008). However, this does not automatically mean that the best course of action is always to offer both. For example, in cases of mild anxiety disorders the American Academy of Child and Adolescent Psychiatry recommends beginning treatment with psychotherapy alone rather than combining with the use of medication (Connolly et al., 2007).

The decision to use medication is a complex one that requires careful consideration of multiple factors, including the severity of symptoms, the degree of impairment caused by the disorder, the level of distress experienced by the child, the potential side effects associated with each medication, and the beliefs held by the patient and family regarding medication. Another factor that will be part of the decision-making process will be the ability and willingness of the child to participate in psychotherapy. For example, a child with severe anxiety causing significant impairment might be highly motivated to participate in treatment and prefer to avoid the use of medication, while a child with only moderate symptoms might be unwilling or unable to do so, making medication a more advantageous option. Or, in another example, a child who is missing school because of school phobia or separation anxiety might require that relatively rapid benefits of medication because of the high degree of impairment inherent in continuously missing school days, even if their level of anxiety and distress would otherwise indicate attempting CBT before introducing medication.

Among the pharmacological agents used in the treatment of anxiety in children, the selective serotonin reuptake inhibitors (SSRIs) are the first line treatments of choice. These medications are generally preferred over the use of treatments such as tricyclic antidepressants, benzodiazepines, or other anxiolytics. SSRIs include a large number of specific medications, and predicting the response of a particular individual to any one of these is difficult. The response of a close relative to a particular medication can sometimes be used as a helpful starting point (for example, if a sibling has done well with one medication it might be tried first). However, sometimes a process of some trial and error will be necessary to determine the medication of choice for a particular child. Although the SSRIs are preferred to the other medications because they are generally well tolerated by children, with few side effects, the effects of long-term use are still insufficiently researched. An important aspect of SSRIs is the time it takes for their effect to be fully actualized. Whereas medications such as benzodiazepines have an almost immediate effect in reducing anxiety, SSRIs generally take between 2 and 4 weeks to take effect. In cases where the use of SSRI has had partial or unsatisfactory results, other medications such as tricyclic antidepressants or neuroleptics can be used to augment the effect of the SSRI.

On pages 298–302 is a table that summarizes the most common medications for each diagnostic category and provides information pertinent to each, including notations for those that have been specifically approved by the FDA for use in children and adolescents. The decision to use medication and the actual implementation should only be carried out in the context of ongoing psychiatric care and management. Child and parents should be provided information on what to expect for both desired effects and side effects and these should be monitored closely, particularly in the early stages of treatment.

Table prepared by Dr. Julie Chilton, MD of the Yale Child Study Center

Disorder	Medication Class	Medication	Issues to Consider
Separation Anxiety Disorder	Selective serotonin reuptake inhibitors	Fluvoxamine	Watch for drug-drug interactions, short half-life
		Fluoxetine	Watch for drug-drug interactions, long half-life, risk of activation
	Tricyclic antidepressant	Imipramine	Poor side effect profile compared to SSRIs, cardiovascular especially
	Benzodiazepine	Clonazepam	Long-acting; watch for withdrawal, disinhibition, sedation, abuse, and dependence
Social Anxiety Disorder	Selective serotonin reuptake inhibitors	Fluvoxamine	Watch for drug-drug interactions, short half-life
		Fluoxetine	Watch for drug-drug interactions, long half-life, risk of activation
		Sertraline	Risk of activation
	Beta blocker	Propranolol	Decrease hyperarousal; monitor cardiovascular side effects
Selective Mutism	Selective serotonin reuptake inhibitors	Fluoxetine	Watch for drug-drug interactions, long half-life, risk of activation

*FDA approved in children and adolescents, varying age limits.

Disorder	Drug Class	Medication	Comments
Obsessive Compulsive Disorder	Selective serotonin reuptake inhibitors	Fluvoxamine*	Watch for drug-drug interactions, short half-life
		Fluoxetine*	Watch for drug-drug interactions, long half-life, risk of activation
		Paroxetine	Short-acting; watch for withdrawal, sedation, drug-drug interactions
		Sertraline*	Risk of activation
		Citalopram	Newer drug, not as much data, few drug-drug interactions, good side-effect profile
		Escitalopram	Newer drug, not as much data, few drug-drug interactions, good side-effect profile
	Tricyclic antidepressant	Clomipramine*	Poor side-effect profile compared to SSRIs, cardiovascular especially
	Partial serotonin agonist	Buspirone	Augmentation of SSRIs, largely anecdotal evidence
Generalized Anxiety Disorder	Selective serotonin reuptake inhibitors	Fluvoxamine	Watch for drug-drug interactions, short half-life

*FDA approved in children and adolescents, varying age limits.

(Continued)

Table prepared by Dr. Julie Chilton, MD of the Yale Child Study Center

Disorder	Medication Class	Medication	Issues to Consider
		Fluoxetine	Watch for drug-drug interactions, long half-life, risk of activation
		Paroxetine	Short-acting; watch for withdrawal, sedation, drug-drug interactions
		Sertraline	Risk of activation
		Citalopram	Newer drug, not as much data, few drug-drug interactions, good side-effect profile
		Escitalopram	Newer drug, not as much data, few drug-drug interactions, good side-effect profile
	Serotonin norepinephrine reuptake inhibitor	Venlafaxine	Watch for diastolic blood pressure elevation at higher doses
	Benzodiazepines	Clonazepam	Watch for withdrawal, disinhibition, sedation, abuse, and dependence
	Partial serotonin agonist	Buspirone	Augmentation of SSRIs, largely anecdotal evidence

*FDA approved in children and adolescents, varying age limits.

Posttraumatic Stress Disorder	Selective serotonin reuptake inhibitors	Fluvoxamine	Watch for drug-drug interactions, short half-life
		Fluoxetine	Watch for drug-drug interactions, long half-life, risk of activation
		Paroxetine	Short-acting; watch for withdrawal, sedation, drug-drug interactions
		Sertraline	Risk of activation
		Citalopram	Newer drug, not as much data, few drug-drug interactions, good side-effect profile
		Escitalopram	Newer drug, not as much data, few drug-drug interactions, good side-effect profile
	Benzodiazepines	Clonazepam	Watch for withdrawal, disinhibition, sedation, abuse, and dependence
	Beta blocker	Propranolol	Decrease hyperarousal; monitor cardiovascular side effects
	Alpha agonists	Clonidine	Decrease hyperarousal; monitor cardiovascular side effects (especially blood pressure) and sedation

(Continued)

*FDA approved in children and adolescents, varying age limits.

Table prepared by Dr. Julie Chilton, MD of the Yale Child Study Center

Disorder	Medication Class	Medication	Issues to Consider
Panic Disorder	Selective serotonin reuptake inhibitors	Fluvoxamine	Watch for drug-drug interactions, short half-life
		Fluoxetine	Watch for drug-drug interactions, long half-life, risk of activation
		Paroxetine	Short-acting; watch for withdrawal, sedation, drug-drug interactions
		Sertraline	Risk of activation
		Citalopram	Newer drug, not as much data, few drug-drug interactions, good side-effect profile
		Escitalopram	Newer drug, not as much data, few drug-drug interactions, good side-effect profile
	Benzodiazepines	Clonazepam	Watch for withdrawal, disinhibition, sedation, abuse, and dependence

*FDA approved in children and adolescents, varying age limits.

Dulcan, M. K., & Lake, M. 2003. *Concise guide to child and adolescent psychiatry* (3rd ed.). Arlington, VA: American Psychiatric.

Walkup, J. T. "Treatment of childhood anxiety disorders," in AACAP's 2012 Psychopharmacology Institute.

Strawn, J. R. 2010. "Diagnosis and treatment of anxiety disorders in children and adolescents," in AACAP's 35th Annual Board Review Course, April 21–24.

References

Connolly, S. D., & Bernstein, G. A., Work Group on Quality I. 2007. Practice parameter for the assessment and treatment of children and adolescents with anxiety disorders. *Journal of the American Academy of Child & Adolescent Psychiatry* 46(2), 267–283.

Walkup, J. T., Albano, A. M., Piacentini, J., Birmaher, B., Compton, S. N., Sherrill, J. T., . . . Kendall, P. C. 2008. Cognitive behavioral therapy, sertraline, or a combination in childhood anxiety. *New England Journal of Medicine* 359(26), 2753–2766.

Family Accommodation Scale – Anxiety (FASA)

DEVELOPED BY:

Eli R. Lebowitz,[a] Joseph Woolston, Yair Bar-Haim,[b] Lisa Calvocoressi,[c] Christine Dauser,[a] Erin Warnick,[a] Lawrence Scahill,[a] Adi Rimon Chakir,[b] Tomer Shechner,[d] Holly Hermes,[a] Lawrence A. Vitulano,[a] Robert A. King,[a] James F. Leckman[a]

[a] Yale Child Study Center
[b] Tel Aviv University School of Psychological Sciences
[c] Yale School of Public Health
[d] National Institute of Mental Health

COPYRIGHT AND PERMISSIONS:

References

Lebowitz, E. R., Woolston, J., Bar-Haim, Y., Calvocoressi, L., Dauser, C., Warnick, E., Scahill, L., Chakir, A. R., Shechner, T., Hermes, H., Vitulano, L. A., King, R. A., & Leckman, J. F. (2012). Family accommodation in pediatric anxiety disorders. *Depression and Anxiety*, 30 (1), 47–54.

Calvocoressi, L., Lewis, B., Harris, M., Trufan, S. J., Goodman, W. K., McDougle, C. J., & Price, L. H. (1995). Family accommodation in obsessive-compulsive disorder. *American Journal of Psychiatry, 152*, 441–443.

Calvocoressi, L., Mazure, C. M., Kasl, S. V., Skolnick, J., Fisk, D., Vegso, S. J., Van Noppen, B. L., & Price, L. H. (1999). Family accommodation of obsessive-compulsive symptoms: Instrument development and assessment of family behavior. *Journal of Nervous and Mental Disease, 187*, 636–642.

Correspondence

Eli R. Lebowitz, Ph.D. Yale Child Study Center: eli.lebowitz@yale.edu

Your name:		Child's name:				
Relationship to child:		Child's age:				

Participation in symptom-related behaviors in the past month

		Never	1-3 times a month	1-2 times a week	3-6 times a week	Daily
1	How often did you reassure your child?	0	1	2	3	4
2	How often did you provide items needed because of anxiety?	0	1	2	3	4
3	How often did you participate in behaviors related to your child's anxiety?	0	1	2	3	4
4	How often did you assist your child in avoiding things that might make him/her more anxious?	0	1	2	3	4
5	Have you avoided doing things, going places, or being with people because of your child's anxiety?	0	1	2	3	4

Modification of functioning during the past month

		Never	1-3 times a month	1-2 times a week	3-6 times a week	Daily
6	Have you modified your family routine because of your child's symptoms?	0	1	2	3	4

(Continued)

Your name:				Child's name:		
Relationship to child:				Child's age:		

Modification of functioning during the past month

	Never	1-3 times a month	1-2 times a week	3-6 times a week	Daily
7	Have you had to do things that would usually be your child's responsibility?	0	1	2	3	4
8	Have you modified your work schedule because of your child's anxiety?	0	1	2	3	4
9	Have you modified your leisure activities because of your child's anxiety?	0	1	2	3	4

Distress and Consequences	No	Mild	Moderate	Severe	Extreme
Does helping your child in these ways cause you distress?	0	1	2	3	4
Has your child become distressed when you have not provided assistance? To what degree?	0	1	2	3	4
Has your child become angry/abusive when you have not provided assistance? To what degree?	0	1	2	3	4
Has your child's anxiety been worse when you have not provided assistance? How much worse?	0	1	2	3	4

Coercive Disruptive Behavior Scale for Pediatric OCD

Coercive Disruptive Behavior Scale for Pediatric OCD (Eli R. Lebowitz, Haim Omer et al., 2011)

Please rate the degree to which the following behaviors characterize your child

	Does your child:	Never	Rarely	Sometimes	Often	Almost all the time
1	Forbid certain actions because of feelings of extreme disgust (e.g., forbids coughing at the table)?	0	1	2	3	4
2	Impose physical closeness or exaggerated clinginess (e.g., won't keep a normal distance, asks never-ending questions)?	0	1	2	3	4
3	Impose strict rules of cleanliness or order on other household members (e.g., demands repetitive cleaning or a special laundry schedule)?	0	1	2	3	4
4	Neglect his/her personal hygiene in a manner that is offensive to others (leaves personal items in public spaces, refuses to shower and smells bad)?	0	1	2	3	4
5	Force you to behave in certain ways or forbid you to do certain things because of extreme pickiness (e.g., forbids certain foods in the	0	1	2	3	4

		0	1	2	3	4
	home, demands specific clothes always be ready)?					
6	Forbid the use of objects in his/her vicinity because of feelings of fear or disgust (e.g., knives, scissors, creams)?	0	1	2	3	4
7	Forbid making changes in the household or react with rage or violence to changes made (e.g., moving furniture, new car)?	0	1	2	3	4
8	Forbid the performance of certain normal actions and activities or react with violence or rage if they are performed (e.g., forbids opening windows or watching TV)?	0	1	2	3	4
9	Force others to make decisions for them or demand endless reassurance to their own decisions?	0	1	2	3	4
10	Perform rituals that cause damage to the surroundings (e.g., ruins items by repetitive cleaning, splashes water over the floors cleaning)?	0	1	2	3	4

(Continued)

Coercive Disruptive Behavior Scale for Pediatric OCD (Eli R. Lebowitz, Haim Omer et al., 2011)

Please rate the degree to which the following behaviors characterize your child

	Does your child:	Never	Rarely	Sometimes	Often	Almost all the time
11	Force others to perform actions on his/her behalf due to feelings of fear or disgust and react to refusal with rage or violence (e.g., to open doors for him because of a fear of touching the handle)?	0	1	2	3	4
12	Demand special "cuddling" or ritualized contact without regard for the will of others?	0	1	2	3	4
13	Forbid the entrance of strangers to the home or limit others in their social activity in the home?	0	1	2	3	4
14	Impose intimacy or act provocatively around others (e.g., walks around naked)?	0	1	2	3	4
15	Repeat actions or words many times and demand that others listen or attend to them until they feel it's enough?	0	1	2	3	4

		0	1	2	3	4
16	Impose physical contact or proximity in a way that is unpleasant to others (e.g., approaches and hugs for a long time, shouts into others' ears)?	0	1	2	3	4
17	Deprive parents or others of sleep (e.g., demands that they be with him all night, turns on and off lights)?	0	1	2	3	4
18	Impose rules or behaviors on others due to tactile or other sensitivity and react to disobedience with rage or violence (e.g., forbids certain sounds, demands specific temperature settings)?	0	1	2	3	4

Author Index

Freeman, J., 40
Freeston, M. H., 78
Friedlmeier, W., 26
Furnham, A. F., 114
Furstenberg, F. F., 281, 282

Garcia, A., 40
Garvey, M., 14
Geffken, G., 39, 40
Geffken, G. R., 15, 38, 260
Gelder, M., 78
Gelder, M. G., 78
Geller, D., 39
Georgiou, G., 55
Gerin, W., 102
Giuliano, P., 282
Glickman, S., 57
Goetsch, V. L., 55
Goldenberg, S., 282, 285
Goldin, P. R., 28
Goldscheider, C., 282
Goldscheider, F. K., 282
Goodman, W. K., 15, 38, 39,
    40, 260, 307
Gorman, J. M., 100
Grabill, K., 15, 38, 260
Greenberg, R. L., 54, 112
Grillon, C., 79
Gross, J. J., 25, 28
Grych, J. H., 235
Guryan, J., 239
Guyer, A. E., 27

Hackmann, A., 78
Harlow, H. F., 142
Harris, M., 38, 307
Hayes, S. C., 77
He, J.-P., 3
Healy-Farrell, L., 41

Hermes, H., 307
Hervey, A. S., 5
Hewitt, P. L., 112
Heyne, D., 275
Hofmann, S. G., 77
Holodynski, M., 26
Hood, J., 235
Hope, D. A., 114
Hsee, C. K., 57
Hudson, J. L., 5, 28
Hurst, E., 239

Jacob, M. L., 15, 38, 260
Janeck, A. S., 28
Janne, P., 281
Jellinek, M. S., 18
Jin, R., 3

Kallen, V. L., 102
Kaplan, L. J., 139
Kashdan, T. B., 114
Kasl, S. V., 307
Kearney, C. A., 269
Kearney, M. S., 239, 269
Kelleher, K. J., 18
Keller, M. B., 4
Kendall, P. C., 296
Kerr, M. E., 141
Kessler, R. C., 3, 10
King, N. J., 275
King, R. A., 307
Kirkcaldy, B. D., 114
Kirshner, M. C., 282
Klein, D. F., 8, 100
Klein, R. G., 100
Kligyte, V., 57
Klumpp, H, 56
Kovalenko, P., 100
Kushner, M. G., 275

Subject Index

321